1,0
HEALTH TIPS

FROM RECENT MEDICAL RESEARCH

EDITED BY
STEPHANIE WIENRICH
& NICHOLAS ALBERY

Published by

The Institute for Social Inventions
20 Heber Road
London NW2 6AA

tel 0181 208 2853
fax 0181 452 6434
e-mail: <rhino@dial.pipex.com>
web: <www.globalideasbank.org>

Further copies of this book are available from the above address for £6.85 incl. p&p. The Institute is grateful to all its correspondents who freely contributed tips for this book, particularly to assistant editor Roger Knights in America. All royalties from this book go to the Institute for Social Inventions' charitable projects (which can be accessed via the web address above). The Institute hopes to bring out an annual edition in future years and urges all those with a concern for the health of their fellow humans to send relevant tips, articles and cuttings (with date and source) to the address above.

Copyright © The Institute for Social Inventions 1998

British Library Cataloguing-in-Publication Data. A catalogue record for this book is available from the British Library.

ISBN 0 948826 50 9

Printed by Esparto Digital Limited, Slack Lane, Derby DE22 3DS

CONTENTS

INTRODUCTION 4
MEN 5
WOMEN 10
   Conception, Pregnancy & Birth 11
   Breast Cancer 14
   The menopause 17
BOTH SEXES 20
   Migraine 20
   Smoking 21
   Heart 22
   Skin 24
   Teeth 26
   Research into HIV and AIDS 27
   Mirror Image Therapy, by Richard Frenkel 29
CHILDREN 31
   Autism 37
FOOD & DIET 39
ALCOHOL 52
   Treating alcoholism 54
DRUGS 57
   Ibogaine 61
LIFESTYLE 64
AGEING 79
   The Attitude Factor 82
   Alzheimer's 92
   Arthritis 96
AND FINALLY... 100
   Health advice online 100
   Twelve warning signs of health 100
INDEX... 101
INSTITUTE PUBLICATIONS 106

INTRODUCTION

Did you know that kiwis are the best fruit to help prevent cancer and heart disease? That selenium has been described as a "birth control pill for viruses"? That DHEA may help boost the ageing immune system? Or that by eating processed tomatoes, you can reduce the risk of prostate cancer?

The 1,001 tips in this book could contribute to the health of every member of the family, from the youngest baby to the eldest grandparent – and should be required reading for every adolescent setting out in life careless of life and limb.

When people are given a diagnosis of cancer or other serious illness, they may suddenly start researching health-promoting diets and other supplements to their medical treatments. But how much more sensible it would be if we all took what simple measures we could to maintain our health throughout our lives, before we have to turn to doctors, hospitals and expensive drugs. After all, it is much easier to sustain our health rather than to try to recover it when it is gone. As one contributor remarked: "Why should anyone with enough money for their basic needs want to win the lottery? If you're healthy, you're already a millionnaire."

> 'Why should anyone with enough money for their basic needs want to win the lottery? If you're healthy, you're already a millionnaire'

This is a book of tips to help keep you on the straight and narrow path of health. But it tries to avoid being a compendium of the latest fads and fancies by focusing on tips which have at least some initial validation from medical or other scientific research.

The reader is defied to read through this book without finding at least half a dozen suggestions that he or she would like to take up immediately. But do check the advice with your doctor, not least because new reseach may render some of the items obsolete.

The suggestions are summarised from literature and cuttings collected over the last seven years by the Institute for Social Inventions in London from correspondents in the UK and the USA, and stored in the Global Ideas Bank on the Internet (www.globalideasbank.org). Wherever the correspondent remembered to provide a date and source, this has also been included.

MEN

- **Unemployed** men who drink **alcohol** are more likely to get jobs than teetotal peers; and the more they drink, the better their prospects. This was the surprising correlation discovered by Employment Services research, and is thought to relate to the **networking** that goes on in pubs (The Times).
- **HRT** may also work for men. Testosterone supplements for middle-aged men, which do carry the risk of exacerbating any prostate trouble, can mitigate the **male menopause** and reduce physical, mental and sexual decline. Research also seems to indicate a role for the hormone in combating heart disease (The Times).
- Proverbial wisdom about **age** telling differently on **men** and **women** has been vindicated by psychiatric research. Declining levels of their respective sex hormones, it appears, tend to produce forgetfulness and confusion in women, while older men become more irritable and impulsive (The Times).
- **Libido** may be a factor in reducing male **longevity**. When marsupial mice are castrated, their lifespan is extended by years, and a study of 319 eunuchs showed their median lifespan to be 13.5 years longer than intact males (New Scientist).

> 'A daily supplement of around 200 micrograms of selenium, also found in brazil nuts, could help protect against cancer and heart disease, and may also boost sperm quality'

- **Finasteride**, drug found in treatments for prostate disease, also appears to be effective in arresting, and in some patients reversing, **hair loss**, but does seem to impair sex drive in some of those who take it (The Times).
- A daily supplement of around 200 micrograms of **selenium**, found in brazil nuts, could help protect against cancer and heart disease, and may also boost **sperm quality** in men. An American study which tracked people on this dosage found cancer incidence reduced by 37 per cent, and overall cancer mortality by 50 per cent (New Age Journal, May 97, monitored for the Institute by Roger Knights). Low levels of selenium in Britain could be contributing to cancers, cardiovascular disease and low fertility levels (The British Medical Journal).
- Men with **symmetrical hands** have **higher sperm counts** than those with digit asymmetry, suggests research carried out an infertility clinic by John Manning at the University of Liverpool. The longer the ring finger is than the index finger also appears to correlate with higher testosterone levels (New

Scientist and The Times, Aug 98).
- Male **infertility** may be helped by taking high-dose **Vitamin E**. When free radicals in the blood react with lipid molecules, they can cause a chain reaction which is thought to damage the sperm membrane. Dr Ford in Bristol is about to begin clinical trials into the action of vitamin E in interrupting this chain reaction (The Times).

'An organic diet was linked to a high sperm density and high sperm count in 30 Danish farmers'

- In a small sample of 30 men, live **sperm counts** were almost double in those whose intake of **organically grown food** was 50 per cent or more (Dr Annette Abell, Department of Occupational Medicine at Aarhus Hospital in Denmark, reported in Planetary Connections, and The Times, 10/6/94: 'An **organic diet** was linked to a high sperm density and **high sperm count** in 30 organic farmers in Denmark, compared to samples from printers, electricians and metal workers').
- Food products which contain **soya** or are wrapped in **plastics**, may **reduce sperm count**, since they contain chemicals which mimic the action of female hormones (Dr Richard Sharpe of the Edinburgh Medical Research Centre for Reproductive Biology).
- The **surfactants** in washing powders, cosmetics and detergents may help cause the fall in men's **sperm counts** (Professor Dennis Lincoln of the Medical Research Council's reproductive biology unity in Edinburgh).
- It is just possible that **alkyl phenols** (one of the breakdown products of detergents, as well as being found in plastics and many other modern products), or **hormones** in the **tap water** we drink, may be responsible for the fact that '**sperm counts** in men have fallen by 50 per cent over the past 30 years, while testicular cancer has risen threefold. Among women, breast cancer has made an ominous but unexplained advance'. However, latest data from British reservoirs (as compared with research done near sewage outfalls on British rivers) is reassuring, and the case remains unproven (The Times, Nigel Hawkes, 30/10/93, reporting on a Horizon programme).
- The antidepressant drug **Anafranil** reduced **premature ejaculation** in a study of 15 men (The Daily Telegraph 30/8/94).
- Men who are **overweight** are 1.4 times more prone to **prostate cancer** than thinner peers, and are likewise more likely to die of it (The Times).
- Men who **dominate** conversations and restlessly compete for attention appear to **die younger** (Journal of the American Psychosomatic Society).
- Men of **higher intelligence** tend also to be **hairier**, according to American research. Hairy chests are apparently more prevalent amongst the

professional classes, and the most intelligent, in a sample of medical students, were more likely to have hairy backs as well (The Times).

• Andy Bryant's remedy for **hair loss** is to stimulate the flow of blood to the head by inverting the body twice a day for a minute or two, to exercise the scalp, face and neck, to reduce stress, to improve diet and to use a shampoo to help open the capillaries. He has coined the acronym **SIDES** to summarise his treatment: stress, inversion, diet, exercise, shampoo. He is claiming an astonishing success rate, with 92 percent of 550 people regrowing their hair (The Independent 27/1/94, an item entitled 'Bristling with confidence' by Andrew Harvey).

• In research which required them to sniff compounds of **hormones** mimicking those secreted at different stages of women's monthly cycles, men showed marked surges in testosterone levels after a noseful of the hormonal cocktail coinciding with ovulation – suggesting an innate ability to **smell** when women are at their most fertile (Sunday Times).

• Men who spend their days sitting at a desk and take little or no **exercise** have at least twice the risk of developing **testicular cancer** than their more active colleagues, according to research published in the British Medical Journal (Jeremy Laurance in The Times).

• Metabolites of **soya protein** and Finnish bread can retard benign prostatic hyperplasia, a condition which is evident in all men to some extent. This could explain why men in the US and the UK are at much higher risk of developing symptoms of **prostatitis** than their counterparts in Finland and the Far East (General Practitioner, 11/10/91, reported in Holistic Health Newsletter).

'Eating tomato products more than twice a week reduced the risk of prostate cancer by up to 34 per cent'

• **Soya beans** could protect men from **prostate cancer**, according to an article in the Lancet that arose from a study of the eating habits of Japanese and Finns. Likewise, soya milk and tofu may protect women against developing breast cancer. The high levels of isoflavonoids in the blood of those on this diet are thought to be a factor, according to Dr David Manning of the Tenovus Cancer Research Centre in Cardiff (Liz Hunt in the Independent, 25/10/93).

• Lycopene, derived in the diet from **tomatoes**, can have health benefits. One large study has shown that those with high levels of lycopene had half the risk of a heart attack and another has shown that eating tomato products more than twice a week, as opposed to never, reduced the risk of **prostate cancer** by up to 34 per cent. Processed tomatoes appears to offer the most benefit

8   1,001 HEALTH TIPS

(tomato sauce, puree and ketchup, but with tomato juice showing little or no benefit). 'Up to 2lbs a day could make all the difference,' says Professor George Truscott, head of the chemistry department at Keele University. Lycopene is also found in watermelon, pink grapefruit and apricots (The Times, 29/5/98).

• **Unripe avocados** contain three related compounds that can kill cancer cells, especially those of **prostate cancer** (New Scientist, 18/7/98).

• Linoleic acid found in **vegetable oils** (used in cereals, snack foods and baked goods) may increase the risk of **prostate cancer**, according to P. A. Godley and colleagues at the University of North Carolina (Aug 97, Positive Health magazine, 51 Queen Square, Bristol BS1 4LH, web: www.positive health.com).

• The average British man waits four years with **prostate** symptoms before getting medical advice. To shorten this delay, a **helpline** staffed by nurses has been set up. Phone Men's Health Matters (London) on 0181 995 4448 on weekdays from 6pm to 10pm (Sunday Times, 10/11/97).

• **Prostatic cancer** claims 11,000 men in the UK each year. In Germany, where Prostatic Specific Antigen blood tests are regularly given, the five-year survival rate is 50 per cent better. Annual PSA testing is needed from the age of 50 (Dr Stuttaford, 'Why early prostate tests are essential', The Times, Jan 98).

• **Selenium supplements** may be useful in treating **prostate cancer** (Positive Health).

• **Saw-palmetto tree berries** have apparently been used to treat **noncancerous prostate enlargement** with twice the success rate of placebos and with fewer side effects than finasteride – a commonly used prescription drug – in a study carried out at the Minneapolis Veterans Medical Centre. However, the results are as yet inconclusive (reported by Brenda Coleman of the Associated Press, 10/11/98).

'Those with a high frequency of sexual intercourse in middle age (45 to 59) had less than half the mortality risk'

• A study in the British Medical Journal (Dec 97) of 918 men living in South Wales found that those with a high frequency of **sexual intercourse** in middle age (45 to 59) had less than half the **mortality** risk of those with a low frequency, as accessed ten years later (Ian Murray, Times report).

• Using a split **bicycle seat** with two sides for each buttock should reduce the reduction in penile sensitivity associated with the pressure placed on the base of the penis by conventional saddles (American journal Sex Over Forty).

• Falls on a bicycle crossbar, parallel bars, horseback, karate kicks – indeed

any damage to the blood vessels of the groin – can cause **impotence** in men (The Times).
- **Nasal decongestants** can cause temporary **impotence**. As can beta-blockers and antidepressants. Doctors should warn their patients (Jane Biddie in The Times, 29/12/92).

'Impotence can be treated with the male equivalent of pelvic floor exercises'

- **Impotence** in some men can be treated successfully with the male equivalent of **pelvic floor exercises**. These lead to a significant improvement in the function of the perineal muscles and so help penile rigidity. The technique is to practise tightening first the back passage muscles, then the front, then both together, whilst sitting, standing or lying down. Count to four slowly, then release. Repeat four times, hourly if possible (The Independent).
- **Smokers** are 1.5 times as likely to suffer **impotence**, even after removing the effects of other possible causes such as drinking, psychiatric problems, heart and circulation problems (American Journal of Epidemiology).
- Research which correlated parental smoking with children's cancer, showed increased risk if the father smoked, but not did not point to greater risk where the mother smoked. This seems to point to **genetic damage** done to **smokers' sperm** (New Scientist).
- A study by the Public Health Institute in Berkeley, California, reviewing 1,000 Finnish men, has found that **despair**, defined as a feeling of "failure or having an uncertain future", led to a greatly increased risk of hardening of the arteries – a cause of **heart disease** and **strokes** (The Times, 2/8/97).
- Men who suppress their anger have a greater risk of developing heart disease, according to a study of 2,500 men. Dealing with angry feelings swiftly and immediately will be less stressful and therefore less damaging to the heart suggests the report (The Times, Sept 98).
- A **ten-minute operation** with a carbon dioxide laser, removing a very small amount of tissue from the soft palate at the back of the throat, can cure **snoring**, without the side effects of conventional palate surgery. (Royal Oldham Hospital, reported in New Scientist 1/4/95).
- Writing in Mims, Dr Hal Yarrow, a retired GP from Hitchin, Hertfordshire says that to cure **snoring** it is best to sleep on the side pressing the elbow into the mattress and using the forearm as a prop, with the chin supported on the back of the hand so as to keep the **chin raised**. His wife reports that since he adopted this position, his own snoring has stopped (The Independent).

WOMEN

- Women can avoid **anxiety** and depression by eating fruit and vegetables – according to a scientist from Wales. Dr David Benton of University College in Swansea studied 1000 people's eating habits to discover that consuming large amounts of **greens** ensures better mental health for women – but not men (The Independent).

> 'Women, but not men, can avoid anxiety and depression by eating large amounts of greens'

- The onset of autumn and winter affects women's moods but not men's, according to researchers from Pennsylvania. A study of more than 1,800 volunteers found that among women, depressive disorders were greatest during autumn and winter, and **anxiety** levels were found to correlate inversely with the amount of **daylight**. No variation was found among men, the researchers said in the British Journal of Psychiatry (Cherrill Hall in The Independent, 28/11/93).
- **Lustral**, one of the group of HT re-uptake inhibitor antidepressants (which also includes the more famous Prozac), seems to be particularly good for sufferers from seasonal affective disorder, or **SAD** (The Times).
- **Light therapy** for SAD sufferers can trigger transient headaches or eye disorders, such as eye strain, seeing spots or blurring (HealthNews, 10/3/98).
- A higher intake of the polyunsaturated fatty acids (pufas) found in **oily fish** may relieve **menstrual pain** (Positive Health).
- Early tests of a mask which flashes red light into the wearer's eyes, and is thought to reset the **body clock** disturbed just before a woman's period, have shown it to reduce the symptoms of **PMT** by 75 per cent (The Observer).
- **Miniskirts** and tight jeans **worn in winter**, by failing to give adequate protection against the cold, promote the growth of thick layers of **fat** on the legs and thighs (The Times).
- Clingy **neoprene sports shorts**, said to promote weight loss, may increase the risk of **blood clots** in the legs (The Times).
- **Exercise** such as one hour's walking a day or two hours' running a week can reduce a woman's risk of **colon cancer** by 46 per cent (Journal of the National Cancer Institute, 2/7/97, monitored for the Institute by Roger Knights).
- **Foods** associated with an increased risk of **cancer** of the lining of the womb are seed oils, butter, sugar, eggs, ham and beef. Vegetables, pasta and fresh fruit halved the risk of the disease, according to a report in Cancer

(quoted by Cherrill Hicks in The Independent).
• The Ortho Tri-Cyclen low dose **birth control pill** has been approved by the American FDA as an **acne treatment** for women over 15 also wanting contraception, helping reduce acne for 80 per cent of participants and often working better than antibiotics or benzoyl peroxide. The pill may also prevent osteoporosis and some cancer (US News & World Report, 10/2/97, monitored for the Institute by Roger Knights).

Conception, Pregnancy & Birth

• Environmental stress has been shown to reduce levels of hormones, and thus of fertility, in female baboons. Since their physiology is very similar to humans, it suggests that **stress reduction** could be a productive treatment for some kinds of human infertility (New Scientist).
• **Egg donors** may risk cancer and infertility, suggests a report of more than 60 studies linking breast and ovary cancer with the fertility drugs used for egg donation (The Observer, 26/7/98).
• Long hours and **stress at work** could put mothers at risk of giving **birth prematurely**, according to research carried out in Italy by Professor Gian Carlo Di Renzo (The Guardian, 9/7/98).
• Smoking **cannabis** could reduce a woman's chances of becoming pregnant. Scientists at the University of Kansas think that its chemical components can inhibit the implanting of an embryo in the uterus walls. There is also evidence that marijuana smoking damages the DNA of unborn children (New Scientist).

'Women who drank at least half a cup of tea a day were more likely to conceive'

• Women who were trying to get pregnant and who drank at least half a cup of **tea** a day were twice as likely to succeed as those who drank no tea, according to researchers at the Kaiser Permanente Medical Care Program in Oakland (New Scientist, Mar 98).
• **Coffee** is suspected of inhibiting conception. Just three cups a day, in a Spanish study, appeared to treble a woman's risk of being infertile, with the heaviest coffee drinkers 45 per cent more likely to take nine months or more to conceive (Sunday Times).
• Women who are **aroused**, enjoy and are satisfied by sexual intercourse are more likely to **conceive**, according to a study of 85 women carried out by Dr Boivin of Cardiff University (The Daily Telegraph and The Guardian, 9/9/98).
• Pregnancy permanently improves the rate at which women clear drugs and **toxins** from their bloodstream, and may reduce the risk of breast cancer

(Daily Telegraph).

• Women with **gum disease** are seven times more likely to give birth to premature, low-birth-weight babies, according to researchers at the University of North Carolina at Chapel Hill (National Enquirer, 11/11/97, monitored for the Institute by Roger Knights).

• A **high temperature** in the early stages of pregnancy, whether from relaxing in saunas or hot whirlpool baths or from fever, doubles the risk of babies being born with neural tube defects such as spina bifida.

• Frequent **ultrasound scans** during pregnancy may result in growth restriction in the womb and the birth of smaller babies, according to a study of almost 3,000 Australian women, reports the Lancet (quoted in an item in the Independent by Liz Hunt, headed 'Ultrasound may harm foetuses').

• Pregnant women or those planning pregnancy should take 0.4mg supplement of **folic acid** daily to reduce the risk of neural tube defects in the foetus, according to a study in the Quarterly Journal of Medicine.

• Women planning to get pregnant can now ask their GPs to prescribe them **folic acid** in order to reduce their chances of having a baby with spina bifida (The Times).

'Women should increase their intake of folic acid to reduce the risk of a child being born with spina bifida'

• All women of childbearing age should increase their intake of **folic acid** to reduce the risk of a child being born with spina bifida or other neural tube defects. Women planning a pregnancy should take a daily 0.4mg folic acid supplement (or 4.5mg daily for women with a spina bifida history) from the start of trying to conceive until the twelfth week of pregnancy, according to the UK's Chief Medical Officer. Folic acid is also found in broccoli, Brussels sprouts, green vegetables, bananas, orange juice, rice, spaghetti, cereals and wholemeal bread (Amanda Ursell in The Guardian; and The Independent, 18/12/92).

• Women with high intakes of **vitamin B6** and **folic acid** also have a 45 per cent lower risk of developing **heart disease** (The Journal of the American Medical Association, reported in The Times, 28/7/98).

• Low-risk pregnant women could do better giving birth at home, but high-risk mothers should go to hospital. Only 2 per cent of women in Britain have **home births** at present, but this number is rapidly rising and Britain has one of the safest records for home births in the world, possibly because pregnant British women are more strictly monitored (British Medical Journal, reported in The Times, 7/8/98).

• Having a **birth companion** reduces your chances of having a Caesarian delivery, as does the choice of a one-to-one midwife over an obstetrician-led team (The Independent).

• Women who have a partner or **midwife** constantly present during labour have less Caesareans and forceps deliveries than those given drugs to speed delivery (British Medical Journal).

• The kind of '**directed pushing**' traditionally encouraged by midwives in women undergoing labour (the Vasalva Method) has no scientific support and may under certain circumstances cause positive damage to the infant and mother – starving the baby of oxygen, and placing undue strain on the woman's vagina. It is generally much healthier for a woman to follow her own intuitive impulses to push (The Independent).

'Healthier for a woman to follow her own intuitive impulses to push'

• **Music therapy** can help with **pain** management during childbirth. Women who listened to music of their choice during labour were half as likely to need anaesthetics, according to a Texan study (reported in Newsweek, 21/9/98, monitored by Roger Knights).

• Babies born in a two-mile radius of **toxic waste** sites have a third higher than average risk of being born with abnormalities. There are currently 400 such licensed sites in Britain (from a study by Helen Dolk from the London School of Hygiene and Tropical Medicine, reported in The Lancet and The Times, 7/8/98).

• Women who began their pregnancy while at the lower end of their recommended **weight-for-height** were three times likelier to have healthy fullterm babies than mothers who were overweight, according to a study of the birth data for 200,000 women by the Karolinska Institute in Stockholm (Sunday Times, 1/3/97).

• Pregnant women who **smoke** may be giving their unborn babies what amounts to a teaspoon of a neat **carcinogen**, according to research carried out at the University of Minnesota Cancer Centre. NNK, a chemical by-product of nicotine, passes through the placenta, and into the foetus' bloodstream, tissues and bone marrow, and could explain why these children tend to go on to develop serious illnesses (The Times, Aug 98).

• **Smokers** who also drink **coffee** when pregnant appear to redouble the risk to their unborn children. Research at St. George's Hospital, London, found that nonsmoking coffee drinkers did not appear to affect the baby's health, but advised women smokers to give up coffee as well as cigarettes while pregnant (The Times).

• A cup and a half of **coffee** per day doubles the risk of miscarriage during the first trimester of pregnancy (Journal of the American Medical Association).

• Pregnant and nursing women who eat from **tin cans** lined with the chemical Bisphenol A may be putting their **male children's health** at risk. The chemical, which can mimic the action of certain human hormones, may lower such men's sperm quality and enlarge their prostate glands in later life (The Independent).

• Pregnant women should wash their hands after contact with a cat, and ensure litter trays are changed regularly, because of the risk of infection with **toxoplasmosis**, a usually subclinical condition which can cause birth defects (The Times). More than 40 per cent of American cats tested carried the bacterium Rochalimaea henselae which in elderly humans, the sick or those with weakened immune systems, can cause lesions of the skin, bone and organs, inflammation of the heart membranes, fever and a condition known as cat-scratch disease – according to the Journal of the American Medical Association (from an item by Liz Hunt in the Independent). The recommendation is that hands should be washed after stroking a cat before preparing any food (Dr Stuttaford in The Times, 3/3/94).

• A follow-up study of the children of participants in a 1950s dietary survey suggests that what women eat during pregnancy can determine their **children's health** in decades to come. Specifically, children of mothers who ate little meat and milk in late pregnancy, or too much sugar in early pregnancy, were likely to suffer high blood pressure in their forties (Sunday Times).

• Pregnant women by eating **bran**-rich food can prevent constipation and thus varicose veins and haemorrhoids (Valerie Yule in a letter to the Institute).

• **Vitamin A** pills, and other supplements high in the vitamin, such as fish liver oil, should be avoided during pregnancy, since increased incidence of **birth defects** is associated with high dosage.

• Delaying the clamping of the **umbilical cord** after premature births by 90 seconds considerably improves the babies' chances, since it allows them to make use of extra blood stored in the placenta (Sunday Times).

• For 42 days after birth, some mothers may wish to abstain from sexual intercourse as there is a risk of death. Before the womb returns to its normal state, air can be forced into blood vessels during sex causing an air embolism and possibly death (The Guardian, 10/1/98).

Breast Cancer

• Regular **exercise**, particularly if taken in the form of a job involving manual labour, appears to reduce the incidence of breast cancer by a third to a half. Excessive exercise does not have the same effect (The Times).

> **'Hormones produced through nipple stimulation may help protect against breast cancer'**

• In a study of 500 women, **exercise** averaging four hours a week since

menstruation reduced the women's chances of developing breast cancer by almost 60 per cent (University of Southern California School of Medicine).
• The hormones produced through **nipple stimulation** (two to three minutes twice a week) may help protect against breast cancer (Prof Tim Murrell, Dept of Community Medicine, University of Adelaide).
• Stretch-material or **sports bras** with sufficient cleavage can prevent or cure lumpy breasts. It has now been found that **benign lumps** in the breast called fibroadenoma are predictors for a greater risk of breast cancer later (Valerie Yule in a letter to the Institute).
• A newly developed test which involves taking **cell samples** from the breast has proved more efficient in detecting the **early stages** of breast cancer than mammography (The Guardian, 10/6/98).

'A new breast cancer screening device uses painless laser imaging technology to create a three-dimensional image of the breast tissue'

• A new breast cancer screening device – computed tomography laser mammography (CTLM) – uses **painless laser imaging** technology to create a three-dimensional image of the breast tissue. It is expected to be far more accurate than a mammogram, and should be available for use in the US from 1999. In the past, many women have complained of the pain and discomfort endured during mammograms and have worried about the effects of X-ray radiation (reported in US News & World Report, 21/9/98, monitored by Roger Knights).
• Women under 45 who have **abortions** have a 50 per cent higher risk of developing breast cancer, according to an American study involving 1,800 women. No increased risk was associated with spontaneous abortion or miscarriage. In Britain, the anti-abortion group Life claims that the risk of developing breast cancer for women who have had an abortion is 30 per cent, but the Royal College of Obstetricians hopes to dispute these claims with their own study (The Independent, 25/10/98).
• **Obesity** greatly increases a woman's risk of getting breast cancer and increases the risk of its being fatal. (Michael Fumento, Reason, April 98, monitored for the Institute by Roger Knights (the reference is to a Nurses Health Study in the Journal of the American Medical Association, Nov 97).
• Air stewardesses may have a greater risk of getting breast cancer because of a **melatonin** deficiency due to jet lag. Melatonin is known to retard the growth of breast cancer cells (The Times, Aug 98).
• **Postmenopausal** breast cancer patients appear to improve their chances of survival if they **stay slim** (The Times).
• Breast cancer tumour-removal operations performed during the **luteal phase** of a woman's **menstrual cycle** (days 0 to 2 and 13 to 32) had the best

outcome, according to a study by Ian Fentiman and colleagues at Guy's Hospital, reported in the British Journal of Cancer (vol 77, p 1502).
• Combining surgery with **chemotherapy**, even when breast cancer has not spread to the lymph nodes, is particularly beneficial for women patients **under fifty**, suggest the findings from a trial run by the Imperial Cancer Research Fund (The Times, Sept 98).
• A new vaccine, **Theratope**, helps women with advanced breast cancer fight the disease by stimulating their immune systems. It also appears to have fewer side effects than chemotherapy (The Times, 10/2/98).
• **Orange juice** made from concentrate blocked breast cancer growth in a study of mice, leading to 50 per cent fewer tumours and metastases than in water-drinking mice (University of Western Ontario, London, Ontario, monitored for the Institute by Roger Knights).
• High **vitamin D** levels aided the survival of women with breast cancer, and could possibly prevent the disease from occurring, according to Prof. Barbara Mawer at the Manchester Royal Infirmary (based on a monitoring of 26 patients). Vitamin D supplements can cause kidney stones in excess, but vitamin D can be acquired naturally from sunlight and from oily fish such as salmon and mackerel (Ian Murray, The Times, 10/2/98).
• A high dietary intake of **calcium** appears to significantly reduce the risk of **kidney stones**, although, paradoxically, the risk actually increases if the calcium is taken in tablet supplements (The Times).
• An article in the Annals of Internal Medicine links **quinine** (the key ingredient in tonic water) to **kidney failure** (Twisted Times #15 94).
• A small American study of 30 recently-diagnosed breast cancer patients showed them to have lower blood levels of **vitamin C**, and to eat **fresh vegetables** less frequently than a control group of healthy women (Positive Health).
• American tests have shown that a naturally-occurring chemical found in **broccoli** cuts the rate of breast cancer in rats. The findings confirm earlier research which showed that a diet rich in vegetables such as broccoli, cabbage and Brussels sprouts reduced the risk of some kinds of cancer (The Times, 12/4/94).

> 'The survival time of women with breast cancer who entered group therapy was twice as long as for those not in therapy'

• The survival time of women with breast cancer who entered **group therapy** was twice as long as for those not in therapy, according to research conducted by Dr David Spiegel of Stanford University (In Context, No. 37, PO Box 11470, Bainbridge Island, WA 98110, USA, tel 206 842 0216; Subs. $31).

Women

- **Cow's milk**, which contains both oestrogen and a potentially carcinogenic peptide known as IGF-I, has been claimed to increase the risk of breast cancer (Washington Physicians Committee for Responsible Medicine).
- **Breastfeeding** for three months or longer can protect a woman against breast cancer, suggests a study in the British Medical Journal. It also suggests that the more babies a woman breastfeeds the less likely she is to get breast cancer. And that roasting and stewing meat and fish are safer than grilling and frying. The latter release substances that may trigger cell mutations in breast tissue, according to a report from Medical World News (The Independent).
- A 26-year old woman taking the contraceptive pill levonorgestrel was prescribed a nasal spray containing the hormone **oxytocin** to help her breastfeed, and felt intense **sexual desire,** two hours after using the spray, for about three hours. Dr Herbert of Cambridge University suggests that the two hormones may act together in a powerful way (British Medical Journal, reported in The Times).

The menopause

- Drinking **alcohol** seems to delay the **menopause**, according to a study of more than 1,000 women aged 45 to 49 by David Torgerson at the University of York (New Scientist, 2/8/97).
- Women who **drink moderately** (5 to 14 units per week) are much less prone to rheumatoid arthritis, particularly if they are postmenopausal (The Times).

'60 per cent of menopausal women taking St John's Wort rediscovered their sex drive'

- In one test, 60 per cent of menopausal women taking Kira, a remedy made from the garden plant, **St John's Wort**, rediscovered their sex drive (Sarah Boseley, The Guardian, 4/11/97).
- **Evening primrose oil** did not help menopausal women with severe hot flushes in a study at the Royal Free Hospital (The Times, 30/3/95).
- **Hormone Replacement Therapy** seems to reduce the incidence of cataracts (American Journal of Epidemiology).
- Women on **HRT** are three and a half times more likely to have an internal blood clot (thrombosis) in their legs. In practice, this means two extra cases in every 10,000 women who take the treatment (The Times).
- On average, the authors of a study of 3000 American women conclude, **HRT** adds 41 months to life-expectancy. Part of this extended longevity may have to do with women who take HRT being generally more health-conscious, but is nevertheless an argument in the treatment's favour (New Scientist, 12/4/97).

- Women on **HRT** appear to have a significantly reduced mortality rate, although this may have to do with healthier lifestyles amongst those taking the treatment (American Journal of Public Health).
- An increased risk of womb cancer in women who have not had hysterectomies is one of the few known drawbacks of **HRT**. This risk, however, can be reduced if the replacement oestrogen is taken in combination with progestogen which latter, unfortunately, is liable to produce some unpleasant mood swings (The Times).
- **HRT** drugs made from the **urine of pregnant mares** (so leading to the slaughter of their foals) are: Premarin, Prempak C, Premique, and Premique Cycle. This would need checking on a regular basis with the manufacturers in case they change their processes. "Other HRT preparations can be taken with an easy conscience by animal-lovers," say the Times (Nov 97).

'Female doctors are five times more likely than their lay patients to use HRT'

- **HRT** tends to return women to their premenopausal hourglass figures (this is often mistaken for weight gain) which in turn helps protect against **heart disease** (Daily Mail).
- Women taking **HRT** are half as likely to lose their **teeth** as other older women, according to an American survey (The Times).
- **HRT** resulted in subtle but significant increases in **intelligence** and memory, particularly with complex tasks, in a study of 36 women (Dr Halbreich at the State University of New York in Buffalo).
- **HRT** may ward off more than hot flushes and brittle bones. If researchers at the University of Southern California are right, women taking oestrogen after the menopause may also reduce the risk of developing Alzheimer's disease, by protecting key cells in the brain (New Scientist, 20/11/93, article by Rosie Mestel entitled 'Can oestrogen fend off Alzheimer's?').
- Anti-inflammatory drugs reduce the risk of developing Alzheimer's disease, while **HRT** is thought to delay the onset of cognitive decline in sufferers (The Times).
- One possible indication of the benefits – on balance – of **HRT**, is that female doctors are five times more likely than their lay patients to use it (British Medical Journal).
- However, a number of leading women doctors have written to the British Medical Journal warning of increased risk of breast cancer, suicide, mood swings and addiction in those taking **HRT** (Independent on Sunday).
- Women on **HRT** may significantly lower their risk of death from colon and rectal cancer (The Wall Street Journal, 5/4/95).
- A study involving 2,027 menopausal women, led by Dr Kristine Ensrud of the Veteran Affairs Medical Center in Minneapolis, found that those taking

only 0.3 milligram of **estrogen** (a low dose form derived from plants and not yet approved for treating osteoporosis or menopausal symptoms) suffered no bone loss and felt fewer unpleasant side effects (Brenda Coleman, Associated Press, 8/12/97).

> 'Estrogen can help maintain skin elasticity, bone strength and protect against heart disease, and it may even protect against Alzheimer's, but it may also increase the risk of breast or uterine cancer by as much as 40 per cent'

Estrogen can help maintain skin elasticity, bone strength and protect against heart disease, and may even protect against Alzheimer's, but it may also increase the risk of **breast or uterine cancer** by as much as 40 per cent. Raloxifene, a so-called **designer estrogen**, seems to offer similar protection against osteoporosis without causing breast or uterine tissue problems, but its long-term effects are not yet known. Raloxifene may act as an anti-estrogen in the brain, and thus could actually increase the risk of developing Alzheimer's, and, because it is related to the cancer drug tamoxifen, could mean that a woman who develops breast cancer while taking Raloxifene could develop tumour cells which are resistant to tamoxifen and thus harder to fight (Time magazine, 1/12/97, monitored for the Institute by Roger Knights).

- Raloxifene, or **Evista**, a drug used to protect women on HRT against **osteoporosis**, may also reduce the risk of breast cancer and lower cholesterol in menopausal women (The Times, 15/9/98).

- Doctors at Jerusalem University confirm the everyday observation that women's skin ages faster than men's. Even premenstrually, women have more **wrinkles** than men, and among the over-60s, women are 75 per cent more wrinkled. However, a study from the Dulwich hospital menopause unit suggests that wrinkling can be stopped and perhaps even reversed by taking **HRT** (The Times, 1/4/93).

- Many skin creams contain alpha hydroxy acids which are thought to alleviate **wrinkles**. These same acids also occur in traditional anti-ageing remedies such as milk, wine and lemons (New Scientist).

1,001 Health Tips, £6.85 incl. p&p from ISI, 20 Heber Road, London NW2 6AA (tel 0181 208 2853)

BOTH SEXES

Migraine

• A **tape recording** of wavelets breaking on a Solway Firth beach has been found to ease symptoms of **tinnitus**, a disabling condition which plagues sufferers with screeches, ticks and whistling noises, quite often stopping them from working and inducing depression. Made by a sufferer from the condition, the gentle wash of sounds on the tape significantly reduces tinnitus symptoms, allowing the sufferer to carry out daily tasks with more ease (The Times).

> 'A tape of wavelets breaking on a Solway Firth beach can ease symptoms of tinnitus'

• Anyone who suffers from **migraines** or **tinnitus**, particularly if the two occur together, would be advised to visit their dentist as these conditions are often associated with teeth grinding, asymmetrical bite and other **dental problems** (British Migraine Association Newsletter, Spring 1997, p. 21).

> 'Headbands with inserts can offer up to 87 per cent pain relief for migraine sufferers'

• **Migraine** sufferers can hold the pain at bay by wearing a tight headband containing inserts (perhaps draughts or backgammon pieces, or just pieces of rubber) placed at points where the pain is most severe. According to a study at the Sacramento Headache and Neurology Clinic the headbands can be worn for up to two hours and seem to work by compressing throbbing blood vessels in the head. The pain may return when the headband is removed, but the study suggests that whilst worn the headbands are up to 87 per cent successful in relieving pain. (The Examiner, 18/5/93).

• A simple **dental splint**, which prevents the wearer from clenching their teeth while sleeping, reduces **migraine** symptoms by 70 per cent, by inhibiting secretions of neuropeptide chemicals (The Times).

• Another, controversial, theory of **migraine**, suggests that it is caused by damage to nerve roots in the upper neck, and can be effectively relieved with a **neck massage** (The Times).

• **Migraine** sufferers should eat regularly and avoid dark alcoholic drinks. The drug **Midrid**, which has recently become available without prescription in the UK, is thought to be effective in relieving the symptoms of migraine, and also of hangovers (The Times).

• In a study of 55 **headache** sufferers at the General Hospital of Luxembourg and in Belgium, it was found that **vitamin B2** (400 milligrams every day for four months) could help the majority to reduce migraine frequency (New Scientist, March 98).

Smoking

• In trials, **smokers** trying to give up doubled their success rates using a **Nicorette Inhalator**, a plastic tube like a cigarette with replaceable cartridges of nicotine (Jeremy Laurance, The Independent, 16/12/97).

• 25 per cent of **smokers** who took an **antidepressant** (bupropion) quit smoking for at least a year – about the same success rate as the nicotine patch (New England Journal of Medicine, reported in Time magazine, 3/11/97, monitored for the Institute by Roger Knights).

• **Cigar smokers** have double the risk of dying from **cancer**, compared with cigarette smokers, according to researchers at the Kaiser Permanente Medical Care Program in Oakland. Chemicals can be absorbed through the mucous membrane in the cheeks (Mandy Payne, Sunday Times).

'Hypnosis is the most effective way of giving up smoking '

• **Hypnosis** is the most effective way of giving up smoking (30 per cent success rate); followed by exercise and breathing therapy (29 per cent); smoke aversion (in which smokers have their own warm, stale cigarette smoke blown back into their faces); acupuncture (24 per cent); nicotine gum (10 per cent); self-help books (6 per cent) (from a meta-analysis covering 72,000 people reported in the New Scientist, 31/10/92).

• People who give up smoking **with other people**, and make use of nicotine replacement products, are up to four times more likely to succeed in kicking the habit (The Independent).

• **Cigarette** smoke may convert **betacarotene** into chemicals which encourage **cancer**. This is the explanation put forward by researchers who have found that heavy smokers appear, contrary to the rest of the population, to increase their risk of lung cancer when taking this antioxidant (New Scientist).

• A study of 29,000 male smokers found a higher incidence of **lung cancer** amongst those who took **betacarotene**. Antioxidant vitamins may have harmful as well as beneficial effects (New England Journal of Medicine).

• **Tobacco** and **alcohol** appear to be even more **carcinogenic** when taken together (The Times).

• **Nicotine** has been shown to have a significant, if short-term, effect in lifting **depression**. Antidepressant drugs may therefore be able to help people kick the habit, by removing what is for many a reason for smoking (The Times).

1,001 Health Tips, £6.85 incl. p&p from ISI, 20 Heber Road, London NW2 6AA (tel 0181 208 2853)

Heart

• To spot a **stroke** with 90 per cent accuracy, have a person lift their arms, squeeze your fingers and smile. This should enable the detection of one-sided motor weakness, a hallmark of a stroke (Time, 24/2/97, monitored for the Institute by Roger Knights).

• A study of residents in Framingham, Massachusetts by a team from Harvard Medical School led by Matthew Gillman has yielded the surprising conclusion that a *reduction* in the risk of getting a **stroke** was linked to *increased* total **fat intake** and to increased consumption of mono-unsaturated fats, such as those found in olive oil – but not to consumption of polyunsaturated fat from fish and vegetables (Nigel Hawkes, The Times, 24/12/97).

• Bananas, spinach, tomatoes and oranges may help guard against **strokes**, as they are all rich in **potassium**. An eight-year study of 440,000 men ranked their potassium intake and found that the top 20 per cent had a 38 per cent lower risk of stroke than the bottom 20 per cent. The top group ate about nine servings of fruit and vegetables a day and smoked and drank less, and exercised more. Potassium supplements, however, can be dangerous in high doses, and should only be taken under the supervision of a doctor (originally published in Circulation, the American Heart Association Journal, and reported in Times Focus, 22/9/98).

• A diet rich in **fish** also helps reduce the risk of dying from a stroke, according to research by Dutch doctors. The group at least risk were those who ate at least 20 grams (7oz) of fish a week.

• Research led by Larry E. Smith of Howard University Hospital in the States, has found that exercise-related **cardiac death** among soldiers was 15 times more likely if the previous day's heat and humidity had reached oppressive levels and had not been followed by rest the following day (Ben Dickinson, Esquire, July 97, monitored for the Institute by Roger Knights).

'10,000 less heart attack fatalities a year if people took aspirin at the onset of chest pains'

• In the USA, about 10,000 deaths a year from **heart attack** could be avoided if people took one 325-milligram **aspirin** at the onset of chest pains (after phoning the emergency service), according to the American Heart Association (Jaime Aron, Associated Press, 21/10/97, monitored for the Institute by Roger Knights).

• People with **heart problems** should take antibiotics an hour before and six hours after going to the **dentist**, to counteract their increased vulnerability to serious bacterial infection (The Times).

• By **donating** three units of **blood** a year a man could possibly reduce the risk of heart disease by reducing the amount of iron in the body (just as menstrual bleeding protects women's hearts). A new study has demonstrated a direct link between heart disease and high iron levels in nearly 2,000 Finnish men (Newsweek, 21/9/92). However, it is worth noting that blood donors are likely to be less at risk of heart attacks anyway because they are more health conscious than non-donors.

'Donating three units of blood a year could lessen the risk of heart disease by reducing the amount of iron in the body'

- **Irregular heartbeat**, which slows down the circulation, also causes tiny blood clots. New research suggests that these cause cumulative damage to the brain, initially impairing memory and concentration and leading on to strokes and dementia. Early treatment with **anti-clotting drugs** could reduce these risks (New Scientist).
- Fat inhibits the ability of coronary arteries to dilate, so **angina** sufferers are much less vulnerable to attacks if they **lower their fat intake**, and up supplements of vitamins C and E (Sunday Times).
- **Betacarotene** containing foods protect against the risk of acute, nonfatal heart attack, concludes a study of women in Northern Italy (Positive Heath, Aug 98).
- Large does of **vitamin E** can give protection against **heart disease**. The protective effect came after people took at least 100mg a day for at least two years. Women then had only half the risk and men a 26 per cent lower risk (Harvard School of Medicine study of 45,270 men and 87,245 women, reported by Celia Hall in The Independent). Vitamin C teams up with vitamin E to prevent LDL cholesterol from sticking to the walls of blood vessels, blocking blood flow and leading to strokes and heart attacks (researcher Lester Packer at the University of California, reported in the Weekly World News, 8/9/92).
- **Sunshine** may cut heart disease – through ultraviolet rays catalysing a reaction which makes vitamin D from one kind of cholesterol. Dr David Grimes in Blackburn has found that the risks of heart attacks are highest in low-altitude and low sunshine areas (Jonathan Foster in The Independent).
- Three or more hours of **brisk walking** a month could protect against heart disease, regardless of genetic predisposition, according to a report in American Medical Association Journal (New Age, Nov/Dec 98, monitored by Roger Knights).
- High doses of **vitamin E** can reduce the risk of a coronary by 75 per cent in patients with **heart disease** (The Lancet).
- Long-term use of decongestant cold remedies could increase the risk of **stroke**, according to a small American study (New Scientist).

1,001 Health Tips, £6.85 incl. p&p from ISI, 20 Heber Road, London NW2 6AA (tel 0181 208 2853)

- Artificial flavours often contain salicylates, a chemical cousin of **aspirin**, which could possibly explain why fewer people in America are dying of heart attacks, according to Lillian Ingster of the National Centre for Health Statistics in Hyattsville (Wall Street Journal, 15/3/96, monitored for the Institute by Roger Knights).
- People drinking more than five cups of **instant coffee** day suffered the least **heart disease** according to a report from Ninewells Hospital in Dundee, in the Journal of Epidemiology (The Independent; and The Guardian 21/6/93). And a 10 year follow-up of 128,800 patients by American researchers has found that people who drank more coffee had a lesser suicide rate. (A similar correlation applied, to a lesser extent, to tea drinkers.) However, a lifetime of drinking two cups of coffee a day increased the level of **osteoporosis** in women, a study in California has found. Researchers estimated that at least one glass of milk a day would have needed to be drunk to compensate for the effect on the bones of these two cups of coffee.

Skin

- Skin specialist Armand Cognetta has had remarkable success in training a dog to sniff out the early symptoms of cancer. Cognetta was inspired to test the possibilities of such an approach after learning that a woman diagnosed with melanoma had first been moved to consult a doctor by the irritatingly persistent interest her dog was showing in the mole on her leg.

'The dog correctly identified malignant tumours in four patients with suspected melanomas'

Working with George, an unusually compliant Schnauzer owned by dog trainer Duane Pickel, Cognetta used samples of cancer cells to attune his senses. Remarkably, George was then able to successfully identify 99 per cent of the cancerous samples presented to him. The dog was then introduced to a number of real patients with suspected melanomas – and correctly identified malignant tumours in four of them. Even more amazingly, George has apparently been able to spot early lung cancer from breath samples.

According to Pickel, this ability stems from a sense of smell 250 million times more acute than humans. This is a rather exaggerated claim, but the general point is borne out by Patrick Riley, Professor of Cell Pathology at University College London. "A large amount of black pigment is produced as a melanoma develops and that creates a smell. We cannot detect the odour, but a dog perhaps can and will find it unpleasant. Their nasal sensory surface is the size of a handkerchief while ours is the size of a postage stamp."

Professor Riley is keen to emphasise the need for extensive testing before becoming too euphoric at this apparent breakthrough. But he is also keen that its potential should be explored as fully as possible: "Typhoid, diabetes and other illnesses have characteristic scents which can be detected by humans in later stages but dogs might be able to identify them earlier."

Further anecdotal evidence for canine diagnostic talents come from Tony Brown-Griffin, who is afflicted with epilepsy. Before acquiring her collie, Rupert, the dangers of fitting had rendered her more or less a recluse, hardly daring to venture out. Luckily, Rupert can apparently scent an impending attack about an hour ahead of its arrival, which he signals by swinging around in front of her and barking. He has also been trained to press a panic button if his owner is left helpless during an attack, which means that she is now able to enjoy a social life again.

Summarised from an article by Beverley Cuddy, entitled 'On the scent of a killer in our midst', in The Mail on Sunday (20/10/96).

'Psoriasis sufferers are travelling to Turkish hot springs to have their skin nibbled by local fish'

• **Psoriasis** sufferers are travelling to Turkey to have their skin nibbled by fish in a hot spring in Kangal (three-week trips cost from £2,500 with Thermalia Travel Ltd, tel 0171 483 1898). A more conventional proven treatment for psoriasis is Aloe Vera.

• A nonprescription cream made from the fatty acids in **banana skins** can help **psoriasis** sufferers by penetrating deep into the skin to reach the infection. The cream, marketed as Exorex, also causes less irritation and is cheaper than leading prescription treatments (The Times, 22/10/98). Exorex helpline: tel 01707 270707.

• Celery that has gone brown is very rich in **psolarens**, which increase light sensitivity, and can cause severe skin reaction in very strong sunlight (The Times).

• **Skin cancer** can now be treated with a new machine which trains **concentrated light** on the affected area, at a fraction of the cost of established laser treatments (The Times).

• Unbleached cotton, certain polyesters and darker or tightly woven fabrics have the highest **sun protection factors**, according to the Skin Cancer Foundation (The Wellness Letter, June 95).

• **Bergamot oil** extracted from the peel of a bitter type of orange, citrus bergamia, grown in the Mediterranean) is found in some sun lotions and has been found to help protect against **skin cancer**, according to the Cancer Research Campaign (Liz Hunt in The Guardian).

• A photodynamic lamp has been successfully used instead of lasers to treat superficial cancers in over 400 patients, reports Colin Whitehurst of the pioneering cancer hospital Christie's in Manchester. It is relatively painless, cheap and quick and has been used to treat 95 per cent of **skin cancers**.

1,001 Health Tips, £6.85 incl. p&p from ISI, 20 Heber Road, London NW2 6AA (tel 0181 208 2853)

Teeth

• Teeth knocked out in sporting activity can be successfully replanted up to 24 hours later, if the tooth is stored in milk (Daily Telegraph).

> 'Teeth knocked out and stored in milk can be replanted up to 24 hours later'

• Frequent **swimming** may turn teeth yellow, as chemicals in the pool can break down proteins in the mouth to form tartar deposits (Sunday Times).
• The gum disease **gingivitis** can be caused by a lack of **folic acid** – the B-complex vitamin found in liver, yeast, fresh fruits and green plants (Alternative Medicine Review, monitored for the Institute by Roger Knights).
• **Gum disease** could be reduced by the use of a toothpaste such as Colgate Total containing **triclosan**, according to a three-year trial with 641 adolescents, led by Prof. Robin Davies at the University of Manchester (Journal of Clinical Periodontology, reported in The Times).
• An antibiotic gel, **atridox**, which can be squirted directly into the bacteria-filled pockets in the gums, could be a painless alternative to root-canal surgery for **periodontal disease** (US News & World Report, 21/9/98, monitored by Roger Knights).
• A new kind of toothbrush, whose fibres can train **laser light** on the teeth, may offer the best oral protection to date. Combined with a special toothpaste, whose action is activated by light, the brush can sterilise the bacteria which cause tooth decay, gum disease and bad breath (New Scientist).
• **Tongue scraping**, or tongue deplaquing, used by the ancient Egyptians and Chinese, is becoming popular again for those with **halitosis** or bad breath. A special scraper which can reach the back of the tongue is being used by dentists and oral hygienists to keep bacteria in check (Seattle Times, 15/7/98, monitored by Roger Knights).
• A series of academic studies has suggested that long-term use of **fluoride** can damage bones, the immune system and the central nervous system. **Fluorosis** can also result (brown staining or fine white lines on teeth enamel). The teeth may even crumble. UK toothpaste manufacturers will now specify fluoride levels on packaging. The BMA does not accept the research findings, but warns against children ingesting too much fluoride (Sunday Times, 15/6/97).
• **Xylitol-sweetened chewing gum** was highly effective in preventing cavities and reversed the early stages of **tooth decay**, according to a 28 month study of 1,227 ten-year olds in Belize carried out by dental researchers at the University of Michigan. Another on-going study of male patients at an Ohio Veterans Administration Hospital suggests the sweetener may be an encouraging treatment for **periodontitis** (the gum disorder that is the chief cause of

tooth loss in adults). The sweetener is produced commercially from birch wood and is similar to Sorbitol and regular sugar, but is chemically different enough to be less likely to promote the growth of decay-causing bacteria.

'Brushing teeth after eating may brush an acidic slurry into the unprotected base of the tooth'

- Brushing your teeth after a meal may be a bad idea – you may brush an acidic slurry into the unprotected base of the tooth, a risk that increases with age. Some dentists advise brushing the teeth before a meal, and **rinsing with water** after eating. Hard cheese eaten at the end of a meal has an anti-caries action; and celery and nuts can help clean the teeth (Times, 18/2/93).
- **Fizzy drinks** and **fruit juices** are best swallowed straight down rather than drunk with a straw or swilled around the mouth, to avoid the acid in the drinks eroding tooth enamel advises the Government's Chief Dental Officer. An average as low as two fizzy drinks a day is associated with **loss of tooth tissue** in children (Shaw et al, British Society of Dental Research).

'Regular wine-tasting can wear away teeth to almost nothing'

- Regular **wine-tasting**, where the acid drink is repeatedly sloshed around the mouth, can wear away teeth to almost nothing (British Dental Journal).
- A team at Guy's Hospital dental school in London have developed a **vaccine** that protects against the bacterium *Streptococcus mutans* that causes **cavities** in the teeth. It could be available from the year 2002, initially through dentists, and later in toothpastes (Nick Nuttall, The Times, 30/4/98).
- A form of bio-active and **bio-compatible glass**, which can be applied in very thin layers like toothpaste, may be an effective protection for **sensitive teeth**. The treatment has been developed by Dr. Leonard Litkowski, director of the bio-active materials and researches programme at the Baltimore dental school at the University of Maryland (The Sunday Times).
- In a three-year experiment, 200 children in Tayside, Scotland, are having their teeth **varnished** with a protective film of Chlorzoin to stop the sugars that cause decay (The Times, 26/4/95).

Research into HIV and Aids

- **Selenium depletion** may speed the progression of HIV infection. Selenium, found in seafood, meat and whole grains, or available as a supplement, may be a future anti-viral agent (Kate Muir, The Times, 30/8/94).
- HIV patients with **low selenium** levels are 20 times more likely to die of Aids than those with normal levels. Low selenium intake has also been linked

to cancer, cardiovascular disease and infertility. Selenium, described as "a birth control pill for viruses" by Will Taylor of the University of Georgia, is found in kidneys, liver, poultry, fish, cereals, and bread made with high protein wheat flour (The Observer, 2/11/97; with additional material from the Telegraph, Ann Kent, 6/3/98).

> 'Selenium, described as a birth control pill for viruses, is found in kidneys, liver, poultry, fish, cereals, and bread'

- Powerful evidence links **antioxidants** not only with a reduced risk of coronary heart disease but also some types of cancer. They almost certainly have a role in a range of other conditions including Parkinson's disease, rheumatoid arthritis, cataracts, some types of male infertility and even Aids.

International experts met at America's National Institute of Health in November 1993 to discuss the possibility that antioxidants found in herbal medicines may prevent HIV being triggered into **full-blown Aids**. The best known antioxidants are betacarotene (the precursor of vitamin A) and vitamins C and E. Back-up troops include the so-called 'scavenger' minerals, selenium, copper, zinc and manganese. Other powerful antioxidants are the polyphenols, found not only in red wine but also in green tea, a staple cholesterol-lowering agent in the traditional Chinese pharmacopeia. Co-enzyme Q10, a polyphenol, is also proving extraordinarily potent at scavenging free radicals. We produce it naturally but stress and nutritional deficiencies deplete our stores, according to Dr Howard Greenspan, an American clinician and researcher (Sarah Stacey in The Sunday Times, 24/10/93).

> 'Aspirin damps down virus replication in HIV-infected tissues (in the test tube)'

- **Aspirin** delays the ageing of tissue (in the test tube); it damps down **virus replication** in HIV-infected tissues (in the test tube); taken regularly it may reduce the risk of colorectal cancer; it adds a health-giving boost to red and white wine; and in small doses it blocks thrombosis and protects against strokes and heart disease (The Guardian, 17/8/94).
- **Mistletoe** contains lectins, viscotoxins and alkaloids which could, according American scientists who have applied to patent its medical use, be extracted to help the body fight both cancer and the HIV virus (New Scientist).
- A 'morning after' pill, or **post-exposure prophylaxis** (PEP), developed for health-workers exposed to the HIV virus, and which uses a combination of the antiviral drugs used to slow the onset of Aids, appears to reduce the risk

of contracting HIV from a needle-prick by 80 per cent. Doctors are hesitant about making it more generally available because of fears that it may undermine safe sex practices (Independent on Sunday).
• A protein in **saliva** protects the white blood cell from infection and means that kissing would not lead to HIV infection (Nigel Hawkes, The Times).
• A **vasectomy** may remove the HIV virus from semen and could help prevent the spread of Aids, according to initial findings by Dr John Krieger at the University of Washington. Examining semen samples from 18 HIV-positive men, he found the virus in 26 per cent of the semen samples but it was not present in any of the semen taken from the four men with vasectomies (Globe, USA, 11/8/92, monitored for the Institute by Roger Knights). Vasectomies, however, increase the risk of cancer of the prostate.

Mirror Image Therapy, by Richard Frenkel

• The mirror is anti-hallucinogenic. When a therapy patient is actively hallucinating, he is asked to look at his image in the mirror and to focus constantly on his image. Invariably the voices disappear from the patient for a period of twenty-one to twenty-six seconds. Ambulatory patients are taught to carry pocket mirrors with them so that they can control the 'voices' any time they wish.

More generally, **Mirror Image Projective Technique** (MIPT) is a diagnostic-therapeutic instrument that is within easy reach of any psychotherapist.

The patient is asked to focus on his mirror image. When the patient becomes inducted into a 'mirror trance', he is then asked to free associate to his image. Defences are unblocked and the unconscious mind is permitted to flow, bringing forth vital feelings and thoughts of recent and past experiences. Intermittently, the patient focuses and unfocuses his eyes upon the image, as he ventures from reality to the unconscious and back. He is a participant observer while using the mirror. In some cases, immediate interpretations can be made from the data gathered. Occasionally, primary instantaneous insight is gained by the patient.

> 'Patients carry pocket mirrors with them so that they can control the voices any time they wish'

Child Mirror Therapy was employed with five child stutterers. The seven-year-old children all took turns using the mirror in the classroom. They free associated to their mirror image rather easily as if it were play therapy. They exposed their problems to their fellow students and teacher. Many simple problems were quickly solved for the children.

Depression. The MIPT is most useful in decreasing depression. The mirror is an antidepressant instrument. At times it will provoke the patient to cry, thus

30   1,001 HEALTH TIPS

relieving anger and reducing the depression in the individual.

Suicide prevention. Since the MIPT decompresses depression, this reduces considerably the chance of the patient acting in a suicidal manner.

Reducing anxiety. The mirror precipitously reduces a patient's anxiety. Mirror responses 'gush out' from the patient and anxiety disappears. I term this the 'gushing phenomenon'. Panic states are thus obviated. Phobic patients are helped by this mirror manoeuvre.

> 'The mirror precipitously reduces a patient's anxiety. Mirror responses gush out from the patient and anxiety disappears. Panic states are thus obviated'

Summarised from the extraordinary volume of 724 pages, The Psychotherapy Handbook, the A to Z Guide to more than 250 Therapies in Use Today *(New England Library, US$ 9-95).*

CHILDREN

- The Maharishi School, which offers **transcendental meditation** and breathing exercises as part of its daily timetable, is top of the Lancashire GCSE league table (all children take at least ten subjects), has won the TES Young Poet of the Week prize more times than any other school, and yet is nonselective in its pupil intake. The school's headmaster, Derek Cassells, argues that this success is due to the twice-daily meditation practised by every pupil (and every teacher).

> 'If you keep children quiet by some form of repression, when the lid comes off – say the teacher leaves the room – the class explodes'

"We want to broaden the debate in education. If you keep children quiet by some form of repression, when the lid comes off – say the teacher leaves the room – the class explodes. We have had a lot of interest from teachers from other schools, who see aspects of our approach that they feel they can use. Even schools that focus purely on academic results, rather than on the children's emotional growth, would benefit from the practice of meditation". The theory behind the practice is that meditation synchronises brain waves, which helps with learning and with creativity. The teachers at the Maharishi School find that their pupils have better concentration, and are more focused and confident than other children; "their minds are settled – which is the source of creativity – and ideas come more readily."

The school was set up by parents in 1986, and now has over 100 pupils aged four to 16. It charges fees, but the teachers and parents raise over £1000 a week to keep these low (about £360 per term) and they hope to open a second school in London in the near future.

Summarised from an article in the Independent. For more information on TM and education, see Teaching Meditation to Children, *by David Fontana and Ingrid Slack, Element, £6.99.*

- Gardens treated with **pesticides** or herbicides are associated with tumours of connective tissues in children, and insecticidal strips in the home with childhood **leukaemia** (New Scientist).
- The burning of Chinese **joss-sticks** releases polycyclic aromatic hydrocarbons, which are linked to contact dermatitis – a marker for increased risk of childhood **leukaemia**, childhood brain tumour and cancer of the nasal passages and pharynx (Bulletin of Environmental Contamination, 97; 57, 361-66, reported in Green World No. 20).

- A study of 2,323 children under ten with **leukaemia** found that the disease correlated with a consumption of more than 12 hot dogs a month. Hot dogs, ham, bacon, sausages, salami and other processed meats contain carcinogenic **nitrites** as preservatives. Vitamin C added to these products can prevent the harmful effect of the nitrites (University of Southern California, reported in The Times).
- Boys who are **short** when they are young are more than twice as likely to be **unemployed** in later life, even if their growth catches up with their peers later on (Journal of Epidemiology and Community Health, August 96).
- **Vitamin A** supplements taken over a three month period speeded **growth** in abnormally short children (those suffering from low levels of growth hormone secreted by the pituitary gland) according to a study from the Hospital Robert Debré in Paris (The Independent Update column).
- Research in China suggests that **zinc** can improve children's growth and intellectual performance, while in Brazil, zinc was shown to improve the immune system in babies (British Medical Journal).
- To avoid microbial contamination, sandwiches for, say, a child's **packed lunch** should be kept at a temperature of below 5 degrees C, in a refrigerator if possible (a chilled insulated bag will take the sandwich up to 10 to 16 degrees). Sandwiches should be kept for the shortest time possible – or be prepared in advance and frozen (John Butters, 'Bacon, listeria and tomato', New Scientist, 9/8/97).
- Breakfast **cereals** and other cereal-rich products like cake mixes, particularly those that have been stored for some time, tend to contain large quantities of microscopic **food mites**, and may help account for the rise in allergic conditions such as **asthma** (Sunday Times).

'Children under two who are given broad-spectrum antibiotics are three times more likely to develop asthma, eczema and hay fever'

- Children under two who are given broad-spectrum **antibiotics** are three times more likely to develop **asthma**, **eczema** and **hay fever** in later life, according to a study of 2,000 patients by Dr Julian Hopkin at Churchill Hospital, Oxford (Louise McKee, The Sunday Times, 1/3/98).
- **Anti-dandruff shampoo** can reduce asthmatic symptoms by increasing breathing capacity by 10 per cent, according to research by five schoolgirls at Cavendish School in Eastbourne. A Brazilian university paediatrics department showed that skin flakes on children's scalps could trigger **asthma** attacks (The Times, 3/11/97).
- Mite-proof covers for pillows, mattresses and duvet, can reduce allergic asthma symptoms by up to 50 per cent, according to research at Southampton

Children

University. Intervent produce the soft breathable plastic with pores too small for the **mite allergen** to penetrate. Allergy to the house dust mite is thought to cause about 80 per cent of **asthma** cases. The textile company Courtaulds has also now developed a pillow for asthma sufferers which contains chemicals that kill the fungi on which the mites feed (New Scientist, 19/9/98). For more details freephone 0800 515 730.

• The mites can also be killed by washing and drying bed linen and placing it in a **deep freeze** for six hours. 'In Scandinavia they hang the bedding out of the window, but here it is seldom cold enough' ('How six hours in a deep freeze can vanquish the British bed bug invasion', by Nigel Hawkes, The Times).

• An American study, meanwhile, has identified another suspected cause of childhood **asthma**: the cockroach. Asthma cases in US cities have grown enormously in 15 years, particularly in the poorer districts where cockroaches are most rife. A study of children hospitalised for an unusually acute strain of asthma showed high numbers of them to be both allergic to cockroaches and to have their droppings and debris in their bedrooms (Seattle Times, monitored for the Institute by Roger Knights).

'Children who bathe every day and wash their hands more than five times are 25 per cent more likely to have asthma'

• The tracking of 14,000 children by the Institute of Child Health at Bristol University has revealed that those children who bathe every day and wash their hands more than five times are 25 per cent more likely to have **asthma** than less clean children, perhaps because the children are exposed to fewer infections and are left more vulnerable and sensitive to allergens (Cherry Norton, Sunday Times, 1/3/98).

• Dietary excess of sodium and Omega-6 fatty acids, and parallel deficiency in antioxidants are also thought to promote the incidence of childhood **asthma**, which has risen dramatically in recent years (Positive Health).

• A 2mg dose of vitamin C taken before exercise appeared significantly to reduce attacks of **asthma** in an Israeli study of young sufferers (Sunday Times).

• Tapes of a **human heart beat** overlaid with soft music help babies – and their parents – sleep more soundly. Terry Woodford has sold over a million copies of his Baby-Go-To-Sleep tapes in the US where they are used by neonatal and intensive care units (for more details call 1-800-537-7748, reported in the National Enquirer, 20/10/98, monitored for the Institute by Roger Knights).

• If newborn babies cannot replace their entire blood supply in the first few days because of haemoglobin problems, **jaundice** and possible brain damage can result. A nurse has now designed a nappy material which lets through **UV light** used in the treatment of such babies, so that they have to spend a third less time under the hot UV lights, but so far her invention is not being mass-produced (New Scientist, Sept 98).

'The risk of cot death is reduced by ensuring babies sleep on their backs with their feet touching the cot end'

- A study of 14,000 infants, led by Dr Peter Fleming of the Institute of Child Health, Bristol University, has found that **babies lying on their backs**, rather than their sides, are less likely to have a wide range of health problems, ranging from coughs and fevers to stomach cramps. The back position has previously been found to be less associated with **sudden infant death** than sleeping face down (Independent, 2/8/97). Research also suggests that babies should have their cots made up with one or more layers of thin blankets well tucked in, with their feet touching the cot end. This discourages them from wriggling down and overheating. **Duvets** and quilts should not be used as these double the risk of cot death for babies in their first year, according to the Department of Health (The Foundation for the Study of Infant Deaths, reported by Ian Murray, The Times, Jan 98).
- Parental **smoking** appears to increase the risk of **cot death** (The Times).
- **Selenium deficiency** may be a significant factor in infant respiratory morbidity.
- Male babies **circumcised** without anaesthetic appear to have their sensitivity to pain increased for months afterward. Even six months later, such babies were shown in tests to react more strongly to the pain of vaccination injections, possibly because they revive memories of the earlier trauma (The Independent).
- According to the Archives of Pediatrics, many mothers do not realise that it may be dangerous to give their babies water in addition to breast milk or formula milk, as babies are unable to **filter water** properly (Time magazine, 1/9/97).
- Some European infant **formula milk** may already be fortified with **LCPUFAs**, fatty acids which promote brain development, after a Scottish study found that babies who had been given the fortified milk scored 'significantly higher' in tests involving finding a hidden toy (Newsweek, 21/9/98, monitored by Roger Knights).
- Trace elements of chlorine compounds called trhalomethanes (THMs) in **tap water** may carry an increased risk of **miscarriage**. Women who are worried about the quality of their local water should consider using a carbon activated filter which removes THMs. Earlier studies suggested an associated increased risk of cancer with THMs (HealthNews, 10/3/98).

1,001 Health Tips, *Institute for Social Inventions, London, 1998, 100pp, ISBN 0 948826 50 9*

- **Babies** can suffer from **cows' milk** protein intolerance. The symptoms can include: nose congestion, snoring, increased mucus flow, bright red cheeks, eczema, sandpaper surface on the face, upper forearms and thighs, frequent coughs and recurrent middle-ear infection (Kathryn Ogg, 'I've had enough of tears before bedtime', Independent, 30/9/97).
- **Breastfeeding** may prevent **schizophrenia** later in life, according to Dr Iain Glen, who heads the Highland Psychiatric Research Group. Researchers at the Craig Dunain Hospital, Inverness, found that over one quarter of patients diagnosed as schizophrenic had levels of essential fatty acid which significantly deviated from the norm. Mother's milk is a far superior source of fatty acid than commercial baby milk powder formulas.

> 'Breastfed babies are less likely to get diarrhoea, ear infections, bacterial meningitis, diabetes, lymphoma and allergies'

- Mothers are recommended to **breastfeed** their babies for at least a year. Breastfed babies are less likely to get diarrhoea, ear infections and bacterial meningitis and are less prone to diabetes, lymphoma and allergies, whilst their mothers gain some protection from ovarian cancer, breast cancer and bone loss in old age (The American Academy of Pediatrics, reported in New Scientist, 13/12/97 and in the Seattle Times, 2/12/97, monitored by Roger Knights).
- In a study of 545 babies, the probability for the development of lung problems was 17 per cent for children exclusively **breastfed** for at least 15 weeks, as against 32.2 per cent for those wholly bottle-fed. The latter also have higher blood pressures (The Times, Jan 98).
- A study of children in Finland suggested that two cups of **coffee** day doubled the risk of **diabetes**, with a higher risk from two cups of tea day (European Journal of Clinical Nutrition).
- Children should not drink more than half a pint of **fruit juice** daily (and perhaps none at all until six months or one-year-old). More can cause **diarrhoea**, whilst being fattening without being nourishing (although high in useful minerals and vitamins). Children should drink juices through a straw so as to protect the **teeth**, and drink the juice later in the day – not after fasting, when it could help give rise to furred-up **arteries** (Dr Stuttaford, The Times, July 97).
- **Chewing gum** sweetened with xylitol, a natural sugar, can reduce **earache** by 40 per cent in children who chew it regularly (The Times).
- Children should be kept away from pets which have been given **anti-flea** treatments, as they are vulnerable to a range of side-effects caused by the chemicals contained in them (The Times).
- Children who eat **fresh oily fish**, very rich in pufas (see above), reduce

their risk of asthma by 75 per cent (New Scientist).
- Children who suffer from **dyspraxia**, a condition producing extreme clumsiness, become much better coordinated if they take supplements of **fish oil**. After supplementation for three months, children in a research group were able to catch a ball for the first time (American Journal of Clinical Nutrition, Winter 96).
- The **daily walk to school** is vital to a child's long-term health and fitness, but nowadays only 59 per cent of primary school children are allowed to walk to school as parents increasingly feel safer dropping their child at the school gates (The Times, 7/9/98).
- Long-distance **running** can cause permanent **spinal damage** in children under 12, whose bodies are insufficiently developed to withstand its strains (The Times).
- Female gymnasts have 20 per cent more bone mass in the lower spine than runners, according to sports scientists at the University of Oregon. Runners had extremely low oestrogen levels, similar to those in postmenopausal women. Low oestrogen may lead to the bone-wasting disease of **osteoporosis**, even in **teenage athletes** (New Scientist).
- Young people, particularly girls, who play a lot of **sport** at school, are much more prone to **delinquent behaviour**, according to a New Zealand survey (The Times).

'Having injections is less painful for children if they pretend to blow bubbles during the ordeal'

- The use of **cotton wool buds** to clean ears often has unpleasant results, a report in Pulse warns. Rex Barton, a specialist at Leicester Royal Infirmary, says that ear wax can become impacted, causing discomfort and loss of hearing. He says parents sometimes are too eager to remove wax from their children's ears. Wax has antibacterial properties, and a normal quantity does not impair hearing (Cherrill Hall in The Independent, 28/11/93).
- Swimming in stagnant lakes in hot weather creates a very high risk of developing **Otitis externa**, an unpleasantly itchy and discharging ear (British Medical Journal).
- Having injections is less **painful** for children if they pretend they are **blowing bubbles** during the ordeal, according to University of Hawaii researcher Gina French. Blowing bubbles relaxes children and gives them something else to think about (monitored for the Institute by Roger Knights).
- Mark Flinn from the University of Missouri has found that children have a threefold increase in the probability of coming down with an upper respiratory infection within seven days of a **high stress event**. (Summarised from an article by Meredith Small entitled 'Bringing up baby' in New Scientist, 24/6/95).

Children

• A study of more than 900 children aged from one to four years, suggested that the more children are **spanked** or otherwise physically punished the lower their scores on **intelligence** tests. This may be partly because those parents who do not spank their children reason with them instead (Murray Strauss of the University of New Hampshire, reported in The Times, 4/8/98).

• Children run an increased **risk of injury** of 1.3 for every hour of **television watching**, according to scientists at the Santa Ana Hospital in Spain. This may be because TV's distorted view of reality affects the way the child relates to its actual surroundings (Journal of the American Medical Association, reported in the Times, August 98).

• New research claims that families that are both "**cohesive**" and "**expressive**" – where conflicts, opinions and feelings are all frequently aired but a strong family bond is sustained – produce higher-achieving children, more resilient to stress (The Times).

• Children, especially boys, who were rated (more than 50 years ago) as prudent, conscientious, truthful and free from vanity lived significantly longer. Childhood cheerfulness and extroversion were inversely related to **longevity**. Children whose parents divorced lived an average of four years less (American Psychologist, reported in The Times, 13/3/95).

Autism

• Autism has not generally been thought of as a condition which responds to treatment, but a treatment pioneered in America is claiming remarkable results; and is being promoted in Britain by **PEACH** (Parents for Early Intervention in Childhood Autism), a new charity. The therapy is intensive, requiring parents to commit at least 30 hours a week over two years, and needs to be undertaken as early as possible, ideally before the child is more than three and a half. But the effort required does seem to pay off. After the treatment, autistic children have achieved previously undreamt-of levels of communication and socialization: the 'unreachable' have been reached.

> 'Give as many rewards for positive behaviour as possible, and avoid punishing'

Lovass treatment, developed by Dr Ivor Lovass, a professor at UCLA, is based around intense and very focused 'behavioural intervention'. Instruction is conducted one-to-one, principally at home, and without distraction from other adults or children. Education, therapy and speech language programmes are broken down in to tiny units, in an individualised tuition programme which stresses the direct involvement of parents, and the careful tailoring of the programme to each child's strengths and weaknesses. One of the important keys seems to be what they call 'non-aversive intervention', where the emphasis is placed on giving as many rewards for positive behaviour as possible, and avoiding punishment. As Lovass puts it, "our goal is to create a joy of learning in children, to make it more fun for them to tune in and learn than to spin or flap or wander around the room ... A cardinal principle is to maximise success, and to make the learning steps easy enough that the child is sure to have a success."

'The first day he worked with a consultant was the first day in his little life he said Yes'

The benefits of the treatment include increased communication, self-help and learning skills. It also seems to reduce the autistic child's characteristically high levels of aggression, self-injury and lethargy. The programme builds up to the point where a child is able to enter mainstream education.

"It was a revelation", says Daniel Hill, whose son Sebastian undertook the programme. "The first day he worked with a consultant was the first day in his little life he said 'yes' ... He now goes to a normal school. The treatment was expensive but more councils are now willing to pay."

The Hills' positive experience with Lovass inspired them to set up the charity, PEACH to promote the treatment. They have plans to establish a centre in London, and are keen to help parents of autistic children to design their own programmes.

Summarised from a story by Carole Woddis, entitled 'He was a different child', in The Independent (8/4/97) and additional information supplied by PEACH (Parents for Early Intervention in Childhood Autism), PO Box 10836, Barnes, London SW13 9ZN.

- Fluvoxamine, an antidepressant marketed as Faverin, appeared to improve behaviour and language use in sufferers from **autism** (Sunday Times).
- There is anecdotal evidence that cutting out **gluten** and **casein** (eg wheat and cow's milk) from the diet, and adding enzymes, vitamins and minerals, can help prevent the damage done by **autism**. Teuvo Rantala, a Finnish nutrition researcher, hypothesises that in some people the peptides resulting from casein and gluten may leak through the brain membrane, damaging the brain's development (John McCrone, New Scientist, 20/6/98).

'Cutting out wheat and cow's milk from the diet can help prevent the damage done by autism'

- **Secretin**, presently only FDA approved as a diagnostic aid for digestive disorders, may help those with autism. A 200-strong parent group in the USA whose children have benefited from the drug is attempting to get the drug's curative powers recognised, but only 20 doctors will administer the drug (The Observer, 13/9/98, monitored for the Institute by Roger Knights).

FOOD & DIET

- Chocolate, especially **dark chocolate**, may help protect against **heart disease**. Like wine, it contains high levels of phenol, a compound which prevents low-density lipoproteins from oxidizing and furring arteries (The Times).
- **Sniffing chocolate** boosts the immune system by encouraging the production of the antibody sIgA, claim scientists from the University of Westminster. The smell of rotten meat caused a drop in the sIgA levels, but the smell of water had no discernable effect (Sunday Times, 8/11/98).
- People who drink three glasses of wine or a pint and a half of beer each day reduce their chances of catching a **cold** – probably because the alcohol reduces stress, which is a major factor in respiratory infections. **Alcohol** was only beneficial for nonsmokers. Of those showing high stress, 50 per cent developed a cold, compared with 22 per cent with low stress (Health Research Unit, University of Wales, reported in The Times, The Independent and The Guardian). Heavy drinking, however, can help cause oral cancer, as can smoking (The Guardian 8/12/92).
- Often-cited medical research discounting **vitamin C** benefit in treating common **colds** may well have been faultily conducted (Positive Health).
- Vulnerability to **cold viruses** amongst those performing heavy physical exercise is considerably reduced by taking **vitamin C** supplements (Positive Health).

> 'Gargling with warm water may be just as effective in treating a throat infection as many antiseptic lozenges and pastilles'

- Gargling with **warm water** may be just as effective in treating a **throat infection** as many antiseptic lozenges and pastilles (Daily Telegraph).
- A couple of glasses of wine or a pint of beer may be a more effective cure for **constipation** than a bowl of bran, and is probably safer than a dose of laxatives says Dr Christopher Probert, a lecturer in medicine at the Gloucestershire Royal Hospital.
- Cancer of the **colon** is associated with diets that are low in calcium, low in dietary fibre and high in fat, according to recent research by Dutch scientists (Dr Derek Gunn in the Brent Recorder).
- Research into the advantages of a high vegetable and low meat diet in preventing **colonic cancer** has not found vitamin supplements to have the same effect as **vegetables** (New England Journal of Medicine).

1,001 Health Tips, £6.85 incl. p&p from ISI, 20 Heber Road, London NW2 6AA (tel 0181 208 2853)

40   1,001 HEALTH TIPS

• Symptoms of **colorectal cancer** to look out for include: blood in the stools, a clear, jellylike mucus around the motions, a change in bowel habit (constipation or diarrhoea), small, narrow stools, loss of weight, unexplained anaemia, pain on going to lavatory or passing wind or a feeling that the bowels are not completely emptied. For further information phone Colon Cancer Concern (London) on 0171 381 4711 (Thomas Stuttaford, 'Check out this stealthy killer', The Times).

• Research by Chris Paraskevan and colleagues at Bristol University suggests that butyrate, derived from **fibre** in the diet, could prevent up to 10,000 cases a year of **bowel cancer** in the UK, if people ate enough fibre for breakfast (Times, 19/11/97).

The findings lend weight to the belief that high-fibre diets – involving cereals, fresh fruit and vegetables – can help prevent **bowel cancers** which are responsible for 20,000 deaths a year in Britain and is the second main cause of cancer death in the industrial world.

• Natural by-products of **high-fibre diets** can cause **bowel cancer** cells to self-destruct. Laboratory experiments at Bristol Medical School have discovered that dietary factors can prompt malignant tumour cell to 'commit suicide' in a natural process which is known as programmed cell death. The researchers also highlighted the key role of naturally accruing fatty acids – the by-product of fibre digestion – in triggering the death of cancer cells (The Guardian, 18/10/93).

• A 53 year-old businessman who ate a portion of **bran** daily for eight months suffered severe small **bowel obstruction** and needed four operations. His surgeon warned the public against overdoing the consumption of bran, despite the benefits of a high-fibre diet (Roger Dobson, 'Good things can be bad', The Independent).

• **Fasting** during the day and eating a large evening meal may raise levels of high density lipoproteins (HDLs) – the good fats which protect against heart disease, according to researchers at Ben Gurion University, Israel (The Independent, reporting a study in the American Journal of Clinical Nutrition).

'Skipping breakfast impairs performance in memory tests'

• However, skipping **breakfast** impairs performance in **memory** tests, according to Dr David Benton of Swansea University in his study of students (The Guardian).

• And **eating frequently** may help you to lose weight, it could be good for your heart and it might, possibly, reduce the risk of diabetes (The Times, 18/2/93).

• John Hopkins University in Baltimore has found that the average diner eats five mouthfuls a minute if **music** with a lively beat is played, four mouthfuls with no music and three mouthfuls if it's a slow melody. They also found that reds, yellows and oranges in the food, plate or decor encouraged diners to **eat more**, as did lingering at festive family occasions (Good Housekeeping, July 97, reported in the Times).

• Steam, grill or bake **aubergine**, as it absorbs more oil than any other vegetable, even potatoes, when fried (The Wellness Letter, June 95).

• A Finnish variety of **margarine** is believed to dramatically reduce blood **cholesterol** levels as plant stanol esters in the margarine stop cholesterol from being absorbed. The brand, Benecol, manufactured by Raisio, will be available for export in 1999, and will be very expensive. The British Heart Foundation also warns that the risk of obesity is not reduced as fat is still absorbed (The Times, 1996, and the Independent, 10/7/98).

• The safest **margarines** for your **heart** are probably Vitaquell, SuperSpread and, to a lesser extent, Flora, as they contain no or less trans-fats. Margarines with trans-fats are linked to heart attacks, according to Dr Albert Ascherio of Harvard Medical School. (Nigel Hawkes in an item in The Times entitled 'Spreading Confusion'.) The linolenic acid in 'high-in-polyunsaturates' margarines such as Flora has, however, been linked to cancerous tumour growth (Barry Groves, Kohima, Lyneham Rd, Milton under Wychwood, Oxfordshire, in a letter to The Times).

• Nu-Trim, a **nutritional soluble fibre fat substitute** made from oats, that carries claims to cut cholesterol levels by up to 10 per cent, is to be on sale in America by the millennium (Times Focus, 25/8/98, monitored for the Institute by Roger Knights).

'Three slices of rye bread a day can cut the risk of death from a heart attack by 17 per cent'

• A **Mediterranean diet** high in fruit, vegetables, olive oil and rape-seed oil margarine which contains an essential fatty acid called alpha-linolenic helped those who had suffered **heart** attacks live longer in a trial by the French National Institute for Health and Medical Research in Lyons (Nigel Hawkes, The Times, 10/6/94).

• Three slices of **rye bread** a day can cut the risk of death from a **heart attack** by 17 per cent. Plant hormones in rye – which is already known to reduce the risk of breast and prostate cancer may be responsible (study of 22,000 men by Finland's National Public Health Institute, monitored by Roger Knights).

• 75 per cent fewer heart attacks were suffered by patients with **heart disease** who were asked to eat more bread, fish, poultry and vegetables, less red meat, to replace butter and cream with margarine and olive oil, and to eat fruit every day. Wine was allowed with meals (Dr Michel Lorgeril and colleagues at The National Institute of Health in Lyons, reported by Jeremy

Laurance in The Times).
• Dr Frederick Stare at Harvard's School of Public Health recommends that we all drink **six to eight glasses of water a day**. Water helps protect the joints from stiffness; can help ward off wrinkles (since good skin tone is dependent on elasticity, which water promotes); can help prevent kidney stones salts may crystallise, forming painful stones, when the kidneys do not get enough water; and drunk before a meal, water aids dieting by filling the belly – plus helping digest the food and pass waste easily, so preventing constipation (from an unidentified American newspaper cutting, 23/11/92, monitored by Roger Knights).
• **Gelatine** (in jellies, Turkish delight, etc) is a pick-me-up that boosts concentration (The Guardian, 22/12/92).
• Creatine, found in **meat**, gives consumers greater reserves of **energy** during exercise and gave competitors in 100 metre and 400 metre events an increase in speed (Nick Nuttall in The Times).
• **Carrots** can be **addictive**, leading to intense withdrawal symptoms, with psychological dependence arising perhaps from the carotene or possibly from some other active ingredient (British Journal of Addiction, reported by Judy Joenes in The Guardian, 1/8/92).
• **Almonds** and **walnuts** reduce **cholesterol** level and may thus help prevent coronary heart disease (American Journal of Clinical Nutrition).
• **Walnuts** are excellent for the **heart**, according to a study from researchers at Loma Linda University, California. They found that a cholesterol-lowering diet which included a moderate quantity of walnuts was more effective than one without (The Independent).
• Eating nuts regularly may protect against coronary heart disease, probably because of their high fibre and polyunsaturated fat content (Californian study reported in Archives of Internal Medicine and The Independent 21/7/92). Amino acids in nuts can help prevent blood clotting, and **linolenic acid** in some nuts – like walnuts – helps protect against heart attacks. Dr Stampfer from Harvard University, says "**Eat more nuts**: it's definitely more beneficial than not doing so, as long as you do more exercise or alter your calorie intake" (The Guardian, 13/11/98).

'For those who ate more nuts on a regular basis, death rates from all causes were cut by almost a quarter'

• In a study of 11,000 volunteers – meat-eaters, semi-vegetarians and vegetarians – over a 13-year period by the University of Otago, New Zealand, and others, it was found that for those who ate more **nuts** on a regular basis, **death rates** from all causes were cut by almost a quarter. Nuts are good sources

of vitamin E, antioxidants, nutrients and linoleic aid (Heart Journal, reported in the Times, 9/11/97).
• **Peanuts** increase cell proliferation in the cellular lining of the **colon** and rectum and thus may be associated with an increased risk of cancer, according to doctors at Northwick Park Hospital and Liverpool University. (The Times, under the heading 'Perilous snack'.)
• Eating at least five servings of **fruit** and **vegetables** a day reduces the risk of breast, lung and colon cancer by up to four times (New Scientist).
• A study of 5,000 **vegetarians** found that they had a 40 per cent lower risk of dying of cancer and 20 per cent lower risk of dying of any cause compared to meat eaters (British Medical Journal).
• 67 per cent of **Belgian pork** contains traces of the sedatives, some banned in Britain, given to the pigs on the way to the abattoir, and 80 per cent of Belgian pork failed hygiene tests by a Belgian consumer organisation (Daily Telegraph, 22/10/98).
• 'Organic' **Swedish pork** may come from pigs fed on meat and bonemeal, a practice banned in the UK (Daily Telegraph, 30/9/98).
• **Spinach** may help **prevent cancer**. Extracts from spinach inhibited the growth of breast and lung cancer cells as well as other carcinogens, according to Dr Shinohara of the national food research institute in Ibaraki, Japan. (The Times, 16/9/92).

> 'It may be possible to treat osteoporosis by a compound containing the fatty acids, GLA and EPA (found in fish oil)'

• **Rape seed oil** cooked at high temperatures gives off carcinogenic compounds, which may account for a correlation discovered in Chinese research between lung cancer and the length of time spent cooking over woks (Shanghai Cancer Institute). And smouldering and burning charcoal from **barbecues** has also been found to emit a range of cancerous airborne chemicals, known as polycyclic aromatic hydrocarbons (PAHs). People who regularly cook on barbecues may be running a risk of **genetic damage** (The Times).
• **Soy sauce** may protect against **cancerous tumours**. Mice fed soy sauce developed far fewer stomach cancers, say researchers at the University of Wisconsin. A mere 25 parts per million of one of soy sauce's flavour agents, HEMF, was sufficient to reduce stomach tumours in mice by 66 per cent (New Scientist).
• Problems with **night vision** associated with dyslexia were found in tests to be relieved by extra fatty acids from fish oil. **Fish oil** taken during pregnancy may also act as a prophylactic against dyslexia in the baby (Jackie Stordy,

University of Surrey, writing in The Lancet).

• **Fish oil** – as distinct from fish liver oil – is thought to be effective in relieving **Crohn's disease**, a disorder of the gastrointestinal tract (New England Journal of Medicine).

• Omega-3 fatty acids of fish and **fish oil** may have a role in the prevention and treatment of **coronary artery disease** after showing composite positive effects in animal, epidemiological and clinical studies (Positive Health, Aug 98).

• It may be possible to treat **osteoporosis** by a new compound containing two **fatty acids**, GLA and EPA, according to the Department of Physiology in Pretoria. Eskimos eat a lot of EPA from **fish oils** (which also help them to avoid kidney stones) The Highland Psychiatric Research Group in Inverness believes that the same GLA and EPA substances may help those schizophrenics who suffer from symptoms of apathy and withdrawal. Dr Horrobin of Scotia Pharmaceuticals is developing a cancer drug, EF13, based on the same principles. It has, in trials, delayed death in patients suffering from pancreatic tumours, and has shown promise against cells infected with HIV. These drugs are said to be completely nontoxic with no side effects (Nigel Hawkes, 'The vast potential of fatty acids', The Times, 9/6/94).

• A highly concentrated form of EPA – found in purified **fish oils** from fatty fish such as salmon, sardines and mackerel – can shrink solid **cancerous tumours** and may halt the dramatic weight loss associated with cancer, according to scientists at Aston University, supported by the Cancer Research Campaign. The latter believe it could explain the low cancer incidence among Eskimos whose diet is rich in fish (The Times, The Guardian and The Independent, 30/12/92).

• Eating mackerel may protect you from **skin cancer**. Research subjects who took 10 capsules of the polyunsaturated fatty acids (pufas) found in **oily fish** over three months gained protection from sunburn equivalent to a factor 3 suncream (The Times).

• **Nutritional guards against cancer** could include: vitamins A, C & E, selenium, zinc, evening primrose oil and fish oils, the co-enzyme Q10 and the mistletoe product Iscador (The Scientific and Medical Network Review).

> 'Humans have a taste for spicy food because spices kill bacteria. Garlic, onion, allspice and oregano kill 100 per cent of bacteria'

• Paul Sharman of Cornell University argues that humans have inherited a taste for spicy food because **spices kill bacteria**. Garlic, onion, allspice and oregano kill 100 per cent of bacteria; Thyme, cinnamon, tarragon and cumin

can kill about 80 per cent, with capsicums, chillies and other peppers killing slightly less (Nigel Hawkes, The Times, 5/3/98).
• Garlic, soybeans, cabbage, ginger, licorice, and umbelliferous vegetables have the highest **anticancer** activity (reports W. Craig from Andrews University, Michigan, reported in Positive Health, Aug 98).
• Freshly pressed **garlic**, even diluted to one part in 250, proved effective against all organisms in a laboratory study, including drug-resistant strains of bacteria (Paediatric Infectious Disease Journal, reported in New Scientist 14/5/94). Garlic also significantly reduced blood cholesterol levels (according to Oxford University's Department of Public Health and Primary Care, reported by Celia Hall in The Independent, under the heading 'Garlic confirmed as heart protector').
• **Garlic** may be an effective treatment for **bladder cancer**. Infected mice injected with garlic extract were shown to have the number of their tumours reduced and their survival rates increased (Sunday Times).

'Kiwi is the most nutritionally dense of the commonly eaten fruit'

• **Iron** supplements may improve **mental performance** (The Times).
• **Dietary iron overload** may contribute to heart disease, cancer, diabetes, osteoporosis and arthritis (Positive Health, 6 Alfred Road, Bristol BS3 4LE, tel 0117 9838851, subs £36). Positive Health is an informative bimonthly magazine, whose editorial content combines insights and research news from both allopathic and 'alternative' – a shorthand term the editors consider pejorative and misleading – medicine. There are regular sections on 'healing', 'bodywork' and approaches to nutrition, amongst other topics. The most interesting part of each issue, however, is a roundup of recent international medical research.
• **Kiwi** is the most 'nutritionally dense' of the commonly eaten fruit – scoring high for vitamin C and E, magnesium, potassium, fibre, serotonin, arginine (used to treat impotence), and nutrients recommended to combat **cancer** and **heart** disease (The Independent, 20/10/97).
• A study, performed by the University of California, studied data from over 11,000 adults ranging in age from 25 to 74 and found that there was a 40 per cent reduction in **risk of death**, especially death caused by cardiovascular disease, in males who had the highest intakes of **vitamin C**. The relationship between vitamin C and cancer was less strong but still indicated possible benefits. The study strongly reinforces other studies that indicate populations consuming diets high in such antioxidants as vitamin C, vitamin E and Beta-Carotene, have lower risks of several chronic diseases (Natural Life USA).
• The Bristol Cancer Help Centre has reviewed over 5,000 medical studies on cancer and diet and in the book Cancer and Nutrition by Dr Rosy Daniel

and Dr Sandra Goodman) they present an overview of the positive scientific evidence, concluding that **cancer** may be prevented by adequate levels of vitamins and minerals. They suggest that it may be wise for those who feel themselves to be at risk of developing cancer to take the following regime: vitamin C (as calcium or magnesium ascorbate) – 500mg tablet three times daily; betacarotene – 6mg tablet two times daily; vitamin E – 133mg (200iu) tablet daily; vitamin B complex – 50mg tablet daily; Selenium 200 microgrammes – one tablet daily. It may also be relevant to take fish oil and linseed oil. (The book costs £6 inc p&p from the Bristol Cancer Help Centre, Cornwallis Grove, Clifton, Bristol BS8 4PG, tel 0117 974 3216.)

• Its role across the spectrum of cancers is debated, but a review of the literature on **vitamin C** suggests that it almost certainly inhibits the development of **gastrointestinal cancers** (Positive Health).

'Sinigrin in Brussels sprouts helps protect against breast, lung and bowel cancer'

• Brussels sprouts contain **sinigrin**, a compound that helps protect against breast, lung and bowel cancer. The sinigrin is particularly rich in the more bitter sprouts (Sunday Times).

• **Vitamin C** may be effective in the treatment of **cancer**. Leicestershire doctor, Dr. Patrick Kingsley, uses 25mg in combination with intravenous oxygen therapy. The **oxygen therapy** fires free radicals at the body, which attack rapidly-reproducing cancer cells, and the vitamin C protects the other cells from oxidative damage. Various other studies have shown that cancer patients taking C have a greater life expectancy (What Doctors Don't Tell You, 4 Wallace Rd., London N1 2PG. tel 0171 354 4592).

• A variety of **carotene** found in tomatoes may have far-reaching effects as a preventative against cancer, heart disease and degenerative eye disease. Lycopene, which is best absorbed by the body when the tomatoes are cooked in virgin olive oil, is the most potent nutritional antioxidant found to date (Daily Mail).

• Evidence that some patients undergoing psychiatric treatment are seriously deficient in **vitamin C** believed to be due in part to an excess of copper in their bloodstream – has led to a variety of experiments with very high doses to see whether it has any therapeutic value in their treatment. Linus Pauling found that those with **schizophrenia** could absorb as much as 40g, suggesting a requirement some 1,000 times the RDA. Dr Allan Cott, New York psychiatrist, treats disturbed children with 2 to 3g of C, in combination with high doses of B vitamins (200mg B5, 150-400mg B6 and high potency B complex.) Dr John Gould has successfully treated alcoholic psychosis and drug withdrawal with intravenous drips containing a similar high-dose mix

(1.5g C, 1g B1, 20mg B2, 200-400mg B3, and 35mg B5) (Organic Living Association Newsletter).

- In a study of 14 patients with **schizophrenia, glycine** – an amino acid found in many foods – was found to lessen withdrawal and confused thinking, although hallucinations and delusions were not affected (American Journal of Psychiatry, Aug 95).
- A simple test which measures **sulphite levels** in **urine** can detect **schizophrenia** at even its earliest stages, claims Dr Soutzos of Guy's and St Thomas' NHS Trust (The Independent, 23/6/98).
- Doctors at the University of Minnesota who carried out research on 759 initially healthy people reported that those with the lowest risk of **heart** disease had the highest levels of **vitamin B6** in the blood. B6 helps produce serotonin (The Times, 28/7/98).
- According to various medical reports, coffee's health effects are not all bad: **caffeine** (found in coffee) can **speed recovery** from a cold, contains antioxidants, can revive a declining memory and can reduce accidents in night workers (The Times, 17/9/97).
- One reason we drink **coffee** may be because it boosts attention and accuracy if drunk regularly when performing repetitive tasks, reports a study on male students at Bristol University (The Times, 22/7/98).

> 'Caffeine is related to theophylline, an asthma medication, and can help relieve a mild asthma attack by opening the airways'

- **Caffeine** is related to theophylline, an asthma medication, and can help with a **mild asthma attack** by opening the airways. About three cups of strong coffee could help with breathing difficulties (see *The People's Pharmacy* book, quoted in the Seattle Times, 15/11/98).
- Jerzy Jankun and colleagues at the Medical College of Ohio in Toledo have argued in Nature that it is the cathechin in **green tea** (available in health stores) which helps prevent **cancer**. The black tea drunk in the West has its cathechins destroyed in the brewing process. Epigallo-cathecin gallate, found in green tea, is a hundred times more effective in soaking up free radicals than vitamin C (Reuters, 5/6/97, and Esquire, Jan 98, an item by Ben Dickinson entitled 'The Organic chemical cocktail', both monitored for the Institute by Roger Knights. And also Health Guardian June 98, reporting on research at Case Western Reserve University School of Medicine that one cup of green tea contains about 200mg of cathechin).
- **Tea** contains an antioxidant chemical, flavonoid, which boosts the body's defence mechanisms against heart attack, according to an article in the Lancet. Apples, onions and red wine also contain **flavonoids**. Drinking green tea has

also been shown to reduce the incidence of cancer of the stomach.
- Drinking both green and black tea which are rich sources of antioxidant **flavonoids**, can help reduce the risk of **major diseases** by counteracting the excess production of free radicals, claims Dr Weisburger of the American Health Foundation. Population surveys have already suggested that those who drink lots of black tea have a lower risk of heart disease (The Guardian, 22/9/98).
- Drinking black tea may also protect against **skin cancer**, since tea contains antioxidants known as **cathechins** which are thought to neutralise the free radicals created by exposure to sunlight (New Scientist).
- **Herpes** may be cured with **old teabags**, preferably Earl Grey, which have been infused in boiling water and then cooled. They should be applied directly onto the herpes sore which should, after four or five days, crust over and disappear (New Scientist).
- High doses of antioxidants such as **vitamin C** could be bad for patients after **cancer** has struck, whilst helping prevent it beforehand, according to research by Jurgen Karzwewski and colleagues at Nijmegen University in Holland (Michael Day, New Scientist, 13/9/97).
- According to biochemists at the University of California, genistein, a substance found in **soya**, weakens the ability of **cancer** cells to grow faster, so they starve and die (Sunday Times).
- Hungry mice on **low calorie diets** developed less **cancer** tumours than those allowed to eat their fill. The same would probably apply to humans, according to a team at the National Institute of Environmental Health Sciences in North Carolina, led by Sandra Dunn (Philip Cohen, New Scientist, 8/11/97).
- A **low-fat diet** appears to slow the spread of non-melanoma **skin cancer** by up to 50 per cent, over the long-term, and to reduce the incidence of keratoses, (noncancerous growths caused by exposure to sunlight) by about 75 per cent (New Scientist).
- A **low-fat diet**, which includes plenty of fibre and vitamin E does seem to reduce the risk of **colon cancer** in the long term (Mutat Res, 19/2/96).
- Research into the effect of **betacarotene** has found that a supplement equivalent to three or four carrots a day significantly increased levels of MHC II molecules in the bloodstream, which are thought to enhance the immune system's ability to identify and act against **cancerous cells** (The Times).
- Antioxidant **vitamins C** and **betacarotene** may prove useful in treating nerve dysfunction associated with **diabetes** (Positive Health).
- The higher the consumption of **carotenes**, the pigment found in orange peppers, green, leafy and yellow vegetables like pumpkins and maize – and particularly the lutein and zeaxanthin carotenes found in dark green leafy vegetables such as spinach – the lower the risk of macular degeneration and

of **blindness** in old age (Journal of the American Medical Association and British Journal of Ophthalmology).

'Antioxidant vitamins such as Betacarotene, C and E, can help delay the onset of cataracts'

- **Antioxidant** vitamins such as betacarotene, C and E, in some cases can delay the onset of **cataracts**, according to research by Dr George Duncan at the University of East Anglia. He recommends a diet high in vegetables such as spinach (The Times, 21/4/94).
- Researchers at Pepsico's research laboratories in Valhalla, New York have found that a **soft drink** with very **high acid content** will **suppress appetite** by between 10 and 30 per cent. Citric and phosphoric acids are blended with still or carbonated water to give a very acid mix. Citrate and phosphate salts are added to buffer the concoction, keeping the pH above 2.5 The sourness is disguised by a hefty addition of glucono-delta-lactone and a dash of artificial sweetener such as saccharine or aspartame. Flavouring the drink with grapefruit juice further masks the acidity (New Scientist, 23/10/93).
- Drinking **water** may be the simplest and cheapest method of **weight reduction** say researchers in Finland. Three-quarters of a pint with breakfast makes people less hungry for the rest of the morning (The Independent).
- Comment from Rodney Aitchey: 'To lose weight very simply, and effectively simply use a **sideplate** instead of the normal full size plate to achieve surprising results after very few days!' (Rodney Aitchey, Y Del, Blaencillech, CastellnewyddEmlyn, Dyfed SA38 9ED Cymru, Wales).
- A **yoghurt** with a creamy emulsion based on a mixture of palm oil and oat oil, developed by Scotia Holdings (UK) but first tried out in Sweden under the name Maval, is said to speed up the natural actions of the small intestine so that **dieters** feel less hungry after eating it than with a normal yoghurt (Paul Durman and Damina Whitworth, The Times, 9/1/98).

'Half of all prescriptions for depression made in Germany are for St John's Wort'

- In tests on 75 obese patients in China, **acupuncture** was shown to have an **anti-obesity** effect and improve water and salt metabolism by regulating the nervous system and body fluid (Positive Health, Aug 98).
- **Acupuncture** seems to improve cellular immune function and may therefore be useful in the treatment of **cancer**. It also had a positive long-term effect on the rehabilitation of **stroke patients** in a study carried out on 45 post stroke patients in Sunnaas Rehabilitation Hospital, Nesoddtangen, Norway (Positive Health, Aug 98).
- Half of all prescriptions for **depression** made in Germany are for St

John's Wort (Hypericum perforatum), a naturally-occurring herb, which numerous studies have shown to be 50 to 80 per cent effective against mild to moderately severe depression (Utne Reader).
- The results of 23 studies on the effects of **St John's Wort** on **depression** show that it is as effective as most prescribed antidepressants without most of the side effects (The British Medical Journal).
- Magnet therapy – or **transcranial magnetic stimulation** (TMS) – which uses a mild magnetic current to stimulate underactive parts of the brain, may offer an alternative to ECT in the treatment of severe depression (Newsweek, 21/9/98, monitored by Roger Knights).
- Because they contain such a wide variety of nutritious chemicals, only some of which can be effectively synthesised into tablet form, **fresh fruit** and **vegetables** eaten regularly are liable to provide greater health benefits than any regime of diet supplements (The Times).
- A high dietary intake of **vitamin C** appears to protect against **gastric cancer**, according to H. M. Zhang and colleagues at the Research Institute International Medical Centre, Tokyo (June 98, Positive Health magazine, 51 Queen Square, Bristol BS1 4LH, web: www.positivehealth.com).
- A Leicester University study of 30 volunteers published in Nature showed that consumption of 500mg a day of **vitamin C** led to a fall of oxoguanine levels in the blood, which could be a sign of an increased risk of **cancer** and heart disease, although levels of protective oxoadenine rose. It took seven weeks for levels to fall back to normal afterwards. Stephen Terrass, technical director of Solgar Vitamins, commented that "this is a single small study, at one dose, over a short time. The results are ambiguous and the conclusions drawn are simply unjustified by the evidence presented" (Nigel Hawkes, The Times, 10/4/98).
- A study of about 10,000 people in Finland, published in the American Journal of Epidemiology, reports that those with the highest consumption of **apples** were less than half as likely to develop **lung cancer** as those who ate few or no apples. This could possibly be due to the antioxidant flavonoids in apples (Jack Broom, Seattle Times, 12/11/97, monitored for the Institute by Roger Knights).

> 'Adults with asthma living in polluted environments could breathe more easily if they took supplements of vitamins C and E'

- Adults with **asthma** living in polluted environments could breathe more easily if they took supplements of **vitamins C** and **E**, according to research at the University of Washington (Sunday Times).
- Higher levels of **magnesium** in the blood – the result of a diet rich in fruit,

vegetables and whole grain – may help prevent **asthma** (Dr John Britton, Nottingham City Hospital).

'19 out of 20 cases of hiccups can be cured by swallowing a teaspoon of sugar'

• 19 out of 20 cases of **hiccups** – including the severe bouts which can last for weeks – can be cured by swallowing a teaspoon of **sugar** (New England Journal of Medicine, monitored for the Institute by Roger Knights).

• **Sugar** mixed with a mild **bacteria-killing iodine** can cure infected wounds (according to an article in The Enquirer).

• The use of **iodised salt** could contribute to **thyroid disease** as surplus iodine can inflame the thyroid. The USA and Japan, who have the highest intake of iodine, also have the highest incidence of chronic autoimmune thyroiditis (The Observer, 9/6/98).

• **Royal Jelly** may actually cause positive harm to asthmatics and others prone to allergy by exacerbating their condition (The Times).

• A study funded by the Scottish Office Agriculture, Fisheries and Environment Department, found that rats feeding on **genetically modified** potatoes for 110 days – equivalent to ten human years – had suppressed **immune** systems. The genes produce proteins called lectins which are known to damage immune-system cells. No GM potatoes have yet been approved for human consumption in Britain (The Times, 10/8/98).

ALCOHOL

- Alcohol **hangovers** may be eased by an amino acid supplement called **N-acetyl-cysteine** (NAC), available from health food shops, according to Carl Waltenbaugh, an alcohol researcher at Northwestern University, Chicago. Some people say that taking one or two grams of NAC clears their head in 20 minutes. (The Times, Dec 97.)
- Milk Thistles contain a chemical – **silymarin** – that inhibits damage to the liver, and could well be an excellent **hangover** remedy (The Times).

'Additives in alcoholic drinks can carry side-effects including nightmares, hyperactivity and itching haemorrhoids'

- Undeclared **additives** in **alcoholic drinks** can carry significant side-effects: nightmares and hyperactivity can be caused by caramel colouring in whisky and in red wine; some ingredients in beers produce itching haemorrhoids; and glycerol in vodka produces anal seepage (letter to New Scientist, 3/5/97).
- Painful **haemorrhoid** flare-ups can be relieved by the use of **nitroglycerin** ointment which causes the muscles in the anal wall to relax, according to the ointment's developer, Dr Gorfine at the Mt. Sinai School of Medicine in New York City (National Enquirer, 20/1/98, monitored for the Institute by Roger Knights).
- The belief that alcohol destroys **brain cells** is being questioned by researchers at the Neurological Research Laboratory in Denmark. They found a reduction in the volume of white matter in the archicortex of dead alcoholics – the archicortex contains the memory centre of the brain. Memory loss is an important symptom of **alcoholic dementia**, but white matter regenerates eventually, if alcoholics stop drinking, whereas neurons do not.
- Contrary to popular belief, beer-drinking does not make you fat. Beer bellies' are acquired because **alcohol stimulates** the **appetite**, and anaesthetises the stomach from feeling full (The Times).
- **Alcohol** with meals **encourages overeating**, by inhibiting the brain's natural calorie-counting centres (American Journal of Clinical Nutrition).
- **Grape juice** can be just as effective as wine in fighting **heart disease** (The Examiner, 18/5/93).
- **Chardonnay** has been suggested to be more beneficial than other wines to people with high cholesterol levels (Linda Bisson of the University of California at Davis).

Alcohol 53

- A large Danish study has shown that a moderate intake of **wine** and **spirits** reduces the likelihood of **peptic ulceration** (Dr Stuttaford, The Times, Dec 97).
- Whisky, drunk neat or with water (and in moderation) reduces the risk of developing **gallstones**. The effect is offset if drunk with a sugary mixer (The Times).
- **Wine drinkers** recovering from operations for **slipped disks** did four times better in the assessments for pain and impairment, two and a half years later, than teetotallers, according to Dr C. Rasmussen of the Hjorring Hospital in Denmark (Thomas Stuttaford, The Times, 30/4/98).
- A survey of medical students found that **vodka** was much more effective in relieving **stress** than red wine (Sunday Times).
- **Heavy drinking** encourages the growth of cancerous tumours (New Scientist).
- Drinking on an **empty stomach** should be avoided by sufferers from **gout** (The Times).
- The use of **mouthwashes** containing **alcohol** could increase the risk of **oral cancer** (Dr John Llewelyn, City Hospital, Edinburgh).
- **Alcohol drinkers** with 'an empty-calorie diet high in white bread and sweets' had a three times higher incidence of **colon cancer** (Journal of the National Cancer Institute).
- **Moderate** consumption of any alcoholic drink not just red wine as was previously thought – can help guard against heart disease. Moderate drinkers are also almost half as likely to suffer from physical and mental ill health as teetotallers, according to research among 9,605 British people born in 1958 (British Medical Journal and The Lancet).

'The fact that moderate drinkers laugh more might explain the supposed health benefits of moderate alcohol intake'

- **Laughter** can boost the **immune system**, and since research shows that moderate drinkers laugh more, this might be the real explanation for the supposed health benefits of moderate alcohol intake. An Australian hospital gave some of its patients regular doses of Fawlty Towers and Billy Connolly and found that laughter not only improved immune function but also provided useful aerobic exercise (The Guardian and Daily Mail).
- For those who would like to receive the supposed benefits of red wine, but don't want to drink alcohol, scientists have extracted the chemicals in **Cabernet Sauvignon** grapes which are thought to act against heart disease, and put them on sale in powder form (The Times).

1,001 Health Tips, £6.85 incl. p&p from ISI, 20 Heber Road, London NW2 6AA (tel 0181 208 2853)

Treating alcoholism

• Joan Mathews Larson, director of the Health Recovery Center in Minneapolis, has developed a **seven-week treatment for alcoholism** that depends on dietary advice and the taking of supplementary vitamins, minerals and other substances.

'Seven Weeks to Sobriety: a seven-week treatment for alcoholism'

Larson, who designed this approach after her son's suicide during treatment for alcoholism, points to published research showing that 74 per cent of her clients remained sober and stable at follow-ups one to three years after treatment, compared with an average of 25 to 30 per cent for other methods.

'One in four deaths among treated alcoholics is suicide'

Researchers have found that abstinent alcoholics normally report feelings of depression, anxiety, psychosis, hostility, paranoia and inadequacy. One in four deaths among treated alcoholics is from suicide; and treated alcoholics have almost the same mortality rate as drinking alcoholics – about three times higher than the general population.

'Alcoholism depletes key antidepressant chemicals in the brain'

Larson believes that alcoholism assaults a person's sanity by depleting key antidepressant chemicals in the brain, a factor which cannot be corrected by counselling alone.

Her programme involves medical assessments, lab tests, the replacement of missing essential elements and aftercare support. At the end of her programme, clients report levels typically 50 per cent lower for aspects such as irritability, depression, poor memory, insomnia, shakiness and exhaustion.

'The formula consists of: glutamine, free-form amino acids, tyrosine, tryptophan, ester C, calcium/magnesium, GLA, a multivitamin/ mineral formula, pancreatic enzymes, betaine hydrochloride, melatonin'

The substances prescribed are many and various, and sometimes in heroic dosages. For instance, the week one 'HRC Detox Formula' consists of glutamine (500mg), free-form amino acids (750mg), tyrosine (800mg), tryptophan (500mg), ester C (675mg), calcium/magnesium (300/150mg), GLA (300mg), a multivitamin/mineral formula, pancreatic enzymes, betaine hydrochloride (648mg), melatonin (time released, 3mg). Later, depending on the patient, other substances, such as DHEA and St John's Wort, may also be advised.

'Long-term dietary advice includes the avoidance of caffeine and sugar'

Larson's book explains how to go about the treatment for those readers unable to attend her centre – although the requirements are so technical that a person would need the backup of a sympathetic doctor and an extremely well-equipped pharmacy (the substances can, however, be ordered from her centre). The centre includes testimonials from satisfied ex-alcoholics such as Jean who writes:

"I followed the book to the letter. I began working out at the YMCA. I began eating healthy. Oh, but it was so tough giving up sugar. I really struggled with that – even more than I did with giving up alcohol. I joined a softball team. I joined a soccer team, and then I met the man that I am currently dating. All the while I was losing weight. Finally, I weighed 116lbs. I started my own business. But the most miraculous thing of all, and most unexpected, was that I no longer have mood swings. None whatsoever! I believe they were all related to sugar and alcohol. My family states that I am not the same person I was for those 15 years."

Seven Weeks to Sobriety *by Joan Mathews Larson, published by Fawcett Columbine of Ballantine Books (1997; ISBN 0 449 00259 4; 335 pages; $12.95). Health Recovery Center, 3255 Hennepin Avenue, Minneapolis MN 55408, USA (tel 612 827 7800); the formulas can be ordered, at least within the States, by phoning 1 800 24 SOBER.*

'Moderation works better than alcohol abstinence'

- Moderation Management and similar treatments in the States are challenging the view that the only way to deal with alcoholism is through total abstinence programmes such as Alcoholics Anonymous and 12-step programmes.

'Abstain for 30 days, and then allow 14 drinks a week'

Moderation Management's guidelines merely require the drinker to abstain for 30 days, and then allow a man 14 drinks a week, with up to four on any one day; and a woman nine drinks a week, with up to three a day.

This approach tends to suit problem drinkers rather than alcoholics – problem drinkers are ones who don't go through withdrawal when they stop; whereas alcoholics exhibit at least three of the following symptoms: drug tolerance, withdrawal, an inability to cut down, sacrificing work, family or social events to drink, devoting a lot of time to finding and consuming alcohol, or persistence in drinking despite health-related problems.

In a 1995 review of treatment programmes, New Mexico psychologists Reid Hester and William Miller found that behavioural measures such as brief interventions, contracts governing drinkers' conduct and coping-skills training, worked better than 12-step programmes of psychotherapy, educational lectures, confrontational counselling and referral to Alcoholics Anonymous.

'Just as in other areas of medicine, least invasive treatments need trying first'

Just as in other areas of medicine, least invasive treatments need trying first, whereas most alcohol treatments start with its most drastic remedy: lifetime abstinence.

Summarised from an article by Nancy Shute, entitled ;The drinking dilemma', in US News & World Report (8/9/97) monitored for the Institute by Roger Knights.

DRUGS

- The British National Formulary (BNF), a bible for GP's which lists every drug on the market, now highlights those drugs that are 'less suitable for prescribing', such as **sudafed**, a commonly used decongestant, and **ferrograd**, a slow-release iron supplement. The cost to the NHS of prescribing drugs which may not be the best, which may not even work, or which may have dangerous side effects, is estimated at £100 million per annum in England alone (adapted from The Guardian, 27/10/98).
- The American drug watchdog (FDA) advises that the following **herbs** should be used with caution, or avoided:

Chaparral, taken to 'purify' the blood, comfrey, for respiratory problems, and Germander, used by dieters, can all cause liver damage; yohimbe, used by bodybuilders, can cause anxiety, seizure, and even death in high doses; lobelia (or Indian tobacco), used by asthmatics, may cause coma or death in high doses; willow bark, often used instead as an analgesic, can have the same side-effects as aspirin (such as stomach problems); and ma huang (or ephedra), taken to boost energy, may cause high blood pressure, nerve damage, or psychosis in high doses (National Enquirer, 24/11/98).

'Aspirin can destroy bowel cancer cells'

- **Aspirin**, already established as a preventative against certain cancers, can actually destroy bowel cancer cells (Independent on Sunday).
- **Aspirin** is now acknowledged not just as a painkiller but as a drug with a variety of uses. A daily aspirin can reduce the likelihood of suffering coronary thrombosis, a transient ischaemic attack (temporary damage to the brain caused by a small blood clot), actual strokes and cataracts. Recently there have been reports that a small daily dose of aspirin reduces the chance of developing cancer of the gastrointestinal tract in general, and the colon, the large bowel and the rectum in particular. Researchers have noted one odd feature in their statistics – if patients prescribed daily drugs for themselves, rather than obtaining them through a doctor's prescription, it seemed that the effect was enhanced (Dr Thomas Stafford, The Times, 1/4/93).
- **Aspirin** also helps protect against nerve cell death. However, aspirin can cause intestinal bleeding and, on occasion, anaphylactic shock in those allergic to it (most often nasal polyps, hay fever and asthma sufferers), as reported in The Times and The Independent.
- Each year, some 7,600 Americans die from **internal bleeding** caused by long-term use of nonsteroidal anti-inflammatory drugs like aspirin. New **supersapirins** – analgesics which block only the enzyme that causes pain and

inflammation, not the version that protects the stomach lining (Cox-2 not Cox-1) – are being developed in the hope that they will have less serious side effects (Time magazine, 13/7/98, monitored by Roger Knights).
• Fasten a slightly wet **aspirin** on to a **wart** with a bandage. Keep the aspirin moist and in place for several days. Once the aspirin is removed, the wart should turn a dark colour and fall off within a week (Privileged Information newsletter, reported in Teleconnect).

'A three-month study testing the effects of shark cartilage on 60 cancer patients in Illinois concluded that it had no effect on their tumours'

• **Squalamine**, a compound found in shark tissue, could well be an effective **anticancer** treatment. By inhibiting the formation of blood vessels to supply tumours, it stops them growing, and is thought to have great potential in preventing regrowth of tumours in postoperative cancer patients (New Scientist).
• The Federal Drug Administration in the States has authorised clinical trials of **shark cartilage**, marketed by a healthfood company in America called Cartilage Technologies under the name Cartilade, to follow up Cuban doctors' claims that the substance causes **cancer tumours** to become smaller or even to disappear. The Cuban work was prompted by the observation of Dr William Lane, an American marine biologist, that sharks rarely suffer from cancer (Sunday Times).
• Although Lane and Comac's book Sharks Don't Get Cancer (1992), suggested that something in **shark cartilage** inhibited angiogenesis which helps feed **cancerous tumours**, the initial research has since been shown to be flawed and trials with interferons or shark cartilage have been halted (The Guardian, 22/9/98). A three-month study testing the effects of shark cartilage on 60 cancer patients in Illinois concluded that it had no effect on their tumours whatsoever – cartilage's advocates found flaws in the study (Times Focus, 30/10/98, monitored for the Institute by Roger Knights).
• **Combretastatin**, a drug made from the bark of the African Bush Willow, can kill **cancerous tumours** by cutting off their blood supply. Tests at Mount Vernon Hospital, Middlesex, have shown remarkable results (Cancer Research, May 97).
• The **immune** systems of patients undergoing surgery for cancer are thought to operate more efficiently if the patient is given an **epidural** rather than a general anaesthetic (New Scientist).
• Drugs derived from a **mould** found growing on a Leeds building site appear to offer a powerful new remedy for dangerous **fungal infections** such as aspergillosis and candida (The Times).

Drugs

- Thrush can be caught from baker's **yeast**, so anyone handling bread or dough is advised to wash their hands thoroughly afterwards (Journal of Clinical Microbiology, July 97).
- In 95 per cent of cases, treatment with **antibiotics** of the bacterium Helicobacter pylori will prevent the formation of **duodenal ulcers** without recourse to the expensive drugs currently used. Antibiotic treatment has the added advantage that it prevents recurrence, unlike many of the more expensive drug treatments currently popular with doctors (The Times, 29/3/93).
- Recent research at Gothenburg University suggests that the symptoms of a cold can be reduced in severity and the attack shortened by taking the anti-asthmatic drug **Intal**, manufactured by Fisons (The Times).

'A report commissioned by the French Health Minister has found marijuana to be relatively harmless, in comparison with alcohol'

- A report commissioned by the French Health Minister has found **marijuana** to be relatively harmless, in comparison with alcohol, which can be as dangerous as heroin and cocaine (New Age, Nov 98, monitored for the Institute by Roger Knights).
- **Marijuana** would be prescribed by nearly half the cancer specialists in America to at least a few of their patients as part of controlling the **side effects of chemotherapy**, if were legal to do so. These were the findings of a MAPS survey of members of the American Society of Clinical Oncology. 63 per cent agreed that it was an effective anti-emetic and 44 per cent had already recommended to at least one patient that they try smoking marijuana. The American DEA continues to claim, however, that marijuana 'has no currently acceptable medical applications', although 13 people in the US may legally smoke it to relieve glaucoma (High Times, Dec 92, monitored for the Institute by Roger Knights. MAPS is c/o Rick Doblin, 1901 Tippah Avenue, Charlotte, NC 28205, USA, tel 0101 704 358 9830; fax 0101 704 358 1650).
- **Cannabis extracts** in pill form can be used to reduce painful muscle spasm. One such modified cannaboid is Zanaflex tizanidine (not recommended for the very young or very old) which causes less drowsiness than other treatments and is used by **Multiple Sclerosis** sufferers (The Times, 11/8/98).
- A component of **marijuana**, cannabidol, seems to be a powerful antioxidant that can help protect brain cells from damage during a **stroke,** and may have some use in the treatment of Alzheimer's and Parkinson's, reports Dr Aidan Hampson at the United States National Institute of Mental Health.

1,001 Health Tips, £6.85 incl. p&p from ISI, 20 Heber Road, London NW2 6AA (tel 0181 208 2853)

- Many millions of people around the world take the antidepressant **prozac** (1 in 6 Americans, according to the Sunday Times) and should be aware that taking this drug (or other serotonin re-uptake inhibitors such as Ecstasy) in conjunction with an MAO inhibitor drug (such as the harmala alkaloids, **Ayahuasca** or analogous mixtures) can result in death (see Neuvonen et al. 1993, Lancet 342 p. 1419). The symptoms are typically initial euphoria, followed by tremors, convulsions and loss of consciousness which can eventually result in death (adapted from an article by J. C. Callaway in MAPS, Spring 94, Newsletter of the Multidisciplinary Association for Psychedelic Studies, subs $40 from MAPS, 1801 Tippah Avenue, Charlotte, NC 28205, USA, tel 704 358 9830; fax 704 358 1650).
- Research by Dr Ricaurte and colleagues seems to show that **Ecstasy** users have long-term nerve damage in the parts of the brain responsible for thought, memory and emotion, and have significantly lower levels of **serotonin** than non-users. Possible effects of this brain damage are depression, anxiety, problems with memory and other neuropsychiatric disorders (The Times, Oct 98).
- Dr George Ricaurte (in a personal communication of 16/11/93 to Nicholas Saunders, the author of *E for Ecstasy*) notes that Ecstasy's toxicity can be prevented by the simultaneous use of prozac fluoxetine, without effecting the experience. Indeed neurotoxicity is prevented even when prozac is taken up to six hours after the MDMA. Dr Ricaurte's research must also cast doubt on the neurological safety of fenfluramine (an appetite suppressant) which has a very similar neurological effect to Ecstasy.
- *In MAPS (Summer 93), Julie Holland writes intriguingly on her view of the potential of a non-neurotoxic future form of MDMA for research purposes:*
It was obvious to me that the research opportunities and possibilities of MDMA were wide open. The potential of this powerful, promising psychotropic seemed limitless: MDMA could be used during any sort of therapy – single, couples, family; as an antidepressant; an analgesic; to facilitate creative visualisation, stress reduction, possibly immune system enhancement; to assist in cognitive restructuring. Who could benefit from a few treatment sessions using MDMA as a chemotherapeutic-adjunct? Who couldn't! What about use in psychosis? In autism? Addiction counselling? As an adjunct to hypnotherapy? I felt like I had just found an 'untapped market'. I was planning on a career in psychopharmacological research and I had found my area of interest.
- Increasing **serotonin** levels (through drugs such as fluvoxamine) can help those suffering from depression, Obsessive Compulsive Disorder, overeating, autism, migraines, premenstrual syndrome and anxiety attacks (Traci Watson, US News & World Report, 25/11/96, monitored by Roger Knights).
- However, increased **serotonin** levels can also increase inflammation of the joints. Antidepressants such as Prozac and Seroxat increase the level of

serotonin and may worsen depressed patients' **arthritis** (The Times, 30/7/98).

Ibogaine

• Promising research with the drug ibogaine – derived from the African Iboga plant – gives hope that heroin and other addictions can be cured – with drugs.

'Early tests show ibogaine to be 70 per cent effective in curing heroin and cocaine addiction'

In 1956 CIBA-Geigy (a major drug company) found ibogaine potentiates morphine analgesia, but did not pursue it. In the early 1960s, American Howard Lotsof, then a heroin addict himself, happened to be offered a dose of ibogaine, with the promise that it would get him really high. He had a remarkable time, seeing visions and being taken back through his personal history, but what really amazed him was that afterwards his desire for heroin had vanished – with no withdrawal pains, and no effort of will.

'Informal' testing amongst addicted friends seemed to confirm Lotsof's findings. Ever since, Lotsof has been campaigning to overcome the American medical establishment's wariness of psychedelic drugs, and have the drug's potential properly researched.

'The average clean period after dosage is about six months'

In 1995, after lengthy indecision, the Federal Drug Administration gave the green light to a series of trials at the University of Miami. It remains to be seen whether their results will back up the growing body of evidence, from drug rehabilitation centres in New York, Panama and Amsterdam, that ibogaine is indeed a potent 'interrupter' of heroin and cocaine addiction. Not surprisingly, the ongoing tests do not show ibogaine as a permanent cure for addiction-but it does seem to offer a reliable, if temporary release from compulsive use. "It's very much determined by who the individual is, what they bring into the treatment, whether they want to stop or whether they're responding to pressure from those around them to stop. Ibogaine is not going to change someone from a person who wants to do drugs into a person who doesn't. But anybody who wants to stop can literally take ibogaine and walk away from drugs," explains Lotsof. In his experience, the average 'clean period' after dosage is about six months. This alone is enough to make it a remarkably successful treatment.

1,001 Health Tips, £6.85 incl. p&p from ISI, 20 Heber Road, London NW2 6AA (tel 0181 208 2853)

Explanations of how it is so effective are harder to come by. Early hypotheses suggest that the drug may achieve its remarkable, painless effects by simultaneously reducing the supply of dopamine, and increasing that of serotonin, to the brain. In this hypothesis, the reduction in the supply of dopamine would both hasten withdrawal and precipitate the characteristic NDE-style visions, whilst the serotonin, known to be associated with feelings of wellbeing, would take the edge off any 'cold turkey'. Other hypotheses emphasise its psychoactive effects, which seems to resemble a kind of intensive psychotherapy.

'Ibogaine allows one to reconfigure the genetic and cultural programming received at birth'

Another interesting, if eccentric, hypothesis about the action of ibogaine was published in 'Green Egg' magazine, by Richard Alan Miller: "Normally the stages of wakefulness of the human brain are: normal waking state, NREM (slow wave or deep sleep), PGO (ponogeniculo-occipital) waves, and REM (rapid eye-movement or paradoxical) sleep. REM sleep is the period when most dreams occur. PGO waves are considered to be the principle coding tool that acts at the cortical level in recording the genetic/epigenetic acquisition necessary for the individuation of the human brain. In other words it is the software-writer aspect of the Self.

"In ibogaine therapy, while the patient is in the near-death dream state, the PGO brain pattern has been found to overlap the standard low alphoid brain state. This precipitates fundamental shifts in instinctual learning patterns, possibly the underlying cause of ibogaine's erasure of addictive behaviour patterns.

"In addition, through random activation mechanisms, PGO waves eliminate from certain types of neuronal networks an informational overload linked to pathological behaviour, thus 'cleaning out' the neuronal circuitry. REM sleep apparently includes a sorting-out and disposal process of the 'residues' stirred up by the PGO wave sleep pattern. The actual dream state could be considered the 're-boot' of the personality rewrite.

"In essence, ibogaine allows one to reconfigure the genetic and cultural programming one receives at birth, much like changing the config.sys file of a computer. The REM aspect then reboots the consciousness patterns with a new autoexec.bat file for habits, needs, and the manner in which one approaches desires."

In the eighties, Lotsof founded a small, private company called NDA International, run out of Staten Island, NY. NDA is developing ibogaine as a treatment to block the physical symptoms of withdrawal from heroin and cocaine. United States patents have been awarded to him as the inventor of the ENDABUSE (Ibogaine) procedure.

Early tests show ibogaine, claims Lotsof, 'to be 70 per cent effective in curing the craving for heroin and cocaine and 100 per cent successful in enabling physical withdrawal'. Most attempted cures for heroin addiction fail 90 per cent of the time.

ENDABUSE is non-narcotic, and not a replacement drug; is non-addicting; is administered orally without injections; is rapid – beginning to work within 35 minutes, and the treatment is completed and the patient sent home within 48 hours; is clinically administered and long lasting – a booster is required in a few cases after 5 or 6 months; and is natural, in that the active ingredient is extracted from the Tabernanthe Iboga plant, found in West Africa (where it is used in rituals related to the Bwiti religion for rites of passage to adult life).

'Drug addiction is an illness of the spirit. You need to do so at that level'

In 1988 doctors in the Netherlands at Erasmus University, Rotterdam, published confirmatory evidence that ibogaine attenuated withdrawal symptoms in rats made morphine dependent (Dzolic, M.R. 1993).

"Ibogaine was used as a rite of passage in Africa," says Lee Hearn, a member of the FDA research team in Miami. "Now it may be used to reprogramme an addict's life. Anecdotal reports indicate that while on ibogaine, he or she is detached from childhood recollection, but coming to grips with it, perhaps for the first time. All neuroses are potentially solvable this way. Drug addiction is an illness of the spirit. If you're going to cure it, you need to do so at that level."

First person accounts from those who have taken the 'ibogaine journey' describe it in even more florid terms: "Now we can resurrect our spirits, re-experience heaven and remember why we came in the first place: to bring our individual facet of heaven here to earth," says one. Another maintains, somewhat mystifyingly, that "I have been held by the Goddess and turning back is not an option."

Summarised from an article by Jerome Burne, entitled 'Is this the valediction to addiction?' in The Independent (2/9/96), from MAPS Vol II No. 1, from an item in Green Action (USA), Vol. 7, No. 1, monitored by Roger Knights, and from a communication from Howard Lotsof. Additional material has been summarised from articles in High Times (Nov 93), Omni (Feb 92), Green Egg (Summer 93), PRL Supplement #7 (Issue No. 8) and MAPS Volume IV, No. 4 (Spring 94) monitored by Roger Knights.

- *Howard Lotsof, NDA International, PO Box 100506, 46 Oxford Place, Staten Island, NY 10310-0506, USA (tel 718 442 2754; fax 201 487 2117).*
- *MAPS, the Multidisciplinary Association for Psychedelic Studies, 1801 Tippah Avenue, Charlotte, NC 28205, USA (tel 704 358 9830; fax 704 358 1650). A website devoted to ibogaine can be found at www.ibogaine.Desk.nl*

LIFESTYLE

• Highly creative persons score both lower and higher than the average person on several scales of such clinical tests as the Minnesota Multiphasic Personality Inventory. Such creative people come out of the test as slightly more 'neurotic' or 'psychotic' on measures of anxiety, depression, schizophrenia and deviance. At the same time, however, they also get high scores for stability and 'ego-strength' – that is, the power to rally from setback and generally cope with adversity.

'The high creatives deliberately challenge and disintegrate themselves'

How can we account for this paradox? How can these people be both crazier and healthier than average?

This apparent contradiction is resolved by the observation that the 'high creatives' deliberately challenge, shake, destabilize, frustrate and disintegrate themselves in order to reassemble the parts better. They know how to set aside control when they need to. To this end they cultivate being both masculine and feminine, logical and emotional, rational and idealistic, excitable and fair-minded, and they move back and forth continuously between such poles.

What about creative therapists? It appears that creative therapists not only do this themselves, but often find ways to put their clients through it too. There seems to be a sort of self-selection of clients, so that the right client gets with the right therapist. There is an ancient belief that when one is ready, one will find the right teacher (from an article by John Rowan in the Newsletter of the Association for Humanistic Psychology, 18a Surrey Road, London, SE15 3AU, tel 0171 732 3481).

• The average systolic blood pressure of **pet owners** was 115 against 135 for non-pet owners; pet owners were more **sociable**, with more contacts with outsiders; and they had closer relationships with their partners – according to a study of 100 couples by Karen Allen of the University of New York at Buffalo, a study part-funded by a pet food manufacturer (Nigel Hawkes, The Times, Mar 97).

'Those with the most diverse social networks had the most protection from the common cold'

• Sheldon Cohen and colleagues at Carnegie Mellon University, in a study of 276 people, found that those with the most **diverse social networks** (with relationships from six or more circles – friends, parents, spouses, neighbours,

work colleagues etc) had the most protection from the **common cold**. Sheer numbers of close relationships did not help (New Scientist, 28/6/97).
• A study by Professor Richard Madeley and colleagues in Nottingham has shown that patients who were not in regular contact with family and friends were 49 per cent more likely to die within three years of a **heart attack**. Having a stressful life, a hard-driving personality or a tendency to depression did not increase the risk. 'There is no doubt that patients with a strong **network of friends** do better than those without,' Professor Madeley said (reported in an article in The Times by Nigel Hawkes entitled 'Keeping busy to survive after heart attack').
• Shy, timid people are more likely to suffer a **cold** than bouncy, outgoing friends, probably, again, because **stress** leads to colds.

'Sex can help ward off colds as it produces immunoglobulin, which is the first line of defence against infection and disease'

• Sex can help ward off **colds**, as it produces a substance called immunoglobulin, which is the first line of defence against infection and disease (the last three items are from Weekly World News, USA, 24/11/92, monitored by Roger Knights).
• Sealing **ventilation** off in winter may well have more to do with seasonal coughs and sneezes than low temperatures (Sunday Times).
• A study of 60 students by Dr Dianne Rice and Roy Baumeister (in Psychological Science) found that **procrastinating students** (who tended to hand work in late) suffered more **colds** and **flu** as term progressed than other students (The Times, Dec 97).
• People with **"enduring social conflicts"** unhappy marriages, miserable jobs, and so on – are more vulnerable to **cold viruses** (The Times).
• **Prolonged stress** may cause permanent brain damage. The stress response activates the HPA axis of the brain, and may eventually damage the brain regions it links (Sunday Times).

'Short-term stress, such as playing a computer game, boosts the ability to fight disease'

• Pessimists get sicker when stressed, while optimists tend to protect themselves from infections. Researchers studying law school students at the University of Kentucky suggest that pessimists can copy the **optimists** and strengthen their **immune systems** with positive thinking when under pressure (New Age, Nov/Dec 98, monitored by Roger Knights).
• Prolonged stress is also thought to weaken the *immune system*. However,

new research suggests that **short-term stress** – such as is experienced while playing a demanding computer game, or making a speech – actually boosts the body's ability to fight disease (The Times).
• Stress may make the brain's protective shield, the blood-brain barrier, more permeable and thus more vulnerable to the action of drugs (Nature Medicine, vol 2, p. 1282).

'Disagreements between couples tend to weaken their immune systems'

• New research at Ohio State University shows that **disagreements** between couples tend to weaken their **immune systems** and make them more susceptible to viruses and even tumours (Kate Muir in an article entitled 'Bicker and you'll get sicker' in The Times).
• Sufferers from **chronic fatigue syndrome** might benefit from a **folic acid** supplement, according to research from Addenbrooke's Hospital in Cambridge (The Independent Update, 15/2/94).
• 200,000 Britons may suffer from **chronic fatigue syndrome** or **ME** (The Times, 17/7/98).
• The physical manipulation and nerve stimulation involved in **massage** can help maintain good health by, among other things, reducing blood pressure, boosting the immune system, raising serotonin levels, and helping with relaxation (Newsweek, 6/4/98, monitored for the Institute by Roger Knights).
• **Self-massage** of the abdomen can relieve **constipation**. A study at the Withington Hospital, Manchester, showed that gentle massage and exercise helped a dozen elderly patients who frequently suffered constipation (The Independent, 13/10/92).

'The high aluminium content of soya milk has begun to worry previously enthusiastic nutritionists'

• Those who had used **aluminium** pots when young ran twice the risk of **brittle bones** and breaking a hip later, according to research at the University of Sydney (Leigh Dayton in the New Scientist, 6/11/93).
• Roll-on deodorants containing **aluminium** can seep into the bloodstream, possibly causing severe health deterioration. Like solvent abuse, inhalant overexposure to deodorants and **antiperspirants** can also cause damage to the internal organs (The International Harry Schultz Letter, and The Times, 5/11/98).
• **Soya milk** has begun to worry previously enthusiastic nutritionists because of its high **aluminium** content (Ethical Consumer).

- Robert Swain and colleagues at the University of Wisconsin have found that the brains of active rats sprouted more capillaries than those of sedentary rats. Swain believes that a similar explosion in capillaries would take place in human **brains** within a month of **physical exercise**, and as a result of mental 'cognitive work-outs', and may protect against age-related decline (Alison Motluk, 'Work-outs keep the brain in shape', New Scientist).

'A 25-minute bout of aerobics made the subjects more creative'

- Middlesex University psychologists studying 63 people who had just completed a 25-minute bout of aerobics found that as well as boosting mood by 25 per cent, the **exercise** made the subjects more **creative** in coming up with unusual uses for everyday objects (Sunday Times, 5/10/97).
- Rats made to run continually on a treadmill had suppressed **immune** system activity compared to rats who could **exercise** when they felt like it, according to researchers at the University of Colorado (Sunday Times, winter 97).

'1mg of vitamin C three times a day will cut the crippling soreness of stiff muscles'

- American researchers have found that those who take 1mg of **vitamin C** three times a day for three days before they start exercising and for seven days afterwards will dramatically cut the crippling soreness of stiff muscles (Pain Journal, reported in The Independent, 3/1192).

'An ounce of brain burns more calories than an ounce of muscle used during exercise'

- An ounce of **brain** burns more **calories** than an ounce of muscle used during exercise. Being conscious is harder work than running to work (Steve Connor in the Independent, reviewing 'The Making of Memory' by Steven Rose, Bantam Press, £16-99).
- **Lack of exercise** increases the chance of cancer of the colon, testes and probably the breast, as well as heart disease (Dr Thomas Stuttaford in The Times, 29/12/92).
- There is some evidence, from a study of **marathon runners**, to suggest that plenty of exercise combined with a low-fat diet actually reduces the body's ability to fight infection (Sunday Times).
- Dr Michael Weintraub, a clinical professor of neurology at New York Medical College, has evidence that **sports** which jolt the body, such as long distance running and high-impact aerobics, lead to **inner ear damage**, with hearing loss at high frequencies, ringing in the ear, dizziness, motion sickness and loss of balance. The daily jolting may displace tiny granules in the inner

1,001 Health Tips, £6.85 incl. p&p from ISI, 20 Heber Road, London NW2 6AA (tel 0181 208 2853)

ear which stimulate the hair fronds that pass sound impulses along the nerves to the brain. The ear damage seems to occur within a few years of starting the exercise, and in one case within less than a year (Kate Muir, 'The Dance of the Deaf', The Times, April 94).

• However, another study suggested that **running regularly boosts enzymes** which help protect against cancer, and counteracts the reduction in such enzymes caused by drinking (New Scientist).

'The life-shortening effects of failing to exercise vigorously are comparable to smoking 20 cigarettes a day'

• The life-shortening effects of failing to **exercise** vigorously are comparable to **smoking** 20 cigarettes a day (a study of 17,300 Harvard graduates, reported by Nigel Hawkes in The Times).

• The severe fatigue which often accompanies **chemotherapy** can be greatly relieved, according to a German study, when patients are given 30 minutes gentle **aerobic exercise** in this instance walking on a treadmill (Sunday Times).

• The Japanese habit of taking **regular stretch breaks** from office routine, rather in the manner that cats and dogs stretch in front of a fire, may help relieve the symptoms of back problems such as **ankylosing spondylitis** (The Times).

• Dr Alan Ebringer of the **Ankylosing Spondylitis** (AS) Research Clinic at the Middlesex Hospital advises his patients to follow a diet low in certain carbohydrates such as potato, bread and flour, especially at times of 'flare-up'. Dr Ebringer needs a minimum of £30,000 a year, a relatively modest amount, to make progress with his dietary research. It seems that orthodox researchers within the establishment control all the purse strings so that innovative approaches are squeezed for funding. Despite several published articles by him on his findings to date, he is denied funding on the grounds of insufficient evidence, when it is only the financing of blood tests etc that would permit this further evidence to emerge. Dr Ebringer argues that people with AS have the tissue type HLA-B27. This resembles the bacteria Klebsiella which normally reside in the bowel. When one eats a large amount of starchy carbohydrate the bacteria feed on it, multiplying in number. In a person with AS this causes inflammation which leads to pain in the joints and lower back. Dr Ebringer believes that there may also be a dietary component in **rheumatoid arthritis**, and that in such cases a high vegetable low meat diet would help – others have also demonstrated this in their research but Dr Ebringer has a complex theory of how this comes about, to do with proteus, the kidneys, urea and the end product of protein metabolism.

Dr Ebringer, AS Research Clinic, The Middlesex Hospital, Arthur Stanley House, 40-50 Tottenham St, London W1P 9PG.

'Stretching exercises to avoid repetitive strain injuries'

- The following are some stretching exercises you can do to avoid repetitive strain injuries or to reduce the inflammation (along with proper work station setup and posture).

(1) Extend your fingers until you feel tension in the stretch. Hold for ten seconds, then bend your fingers at the knuckles (do not clench your fist). Hold this position for ten seconds, then release. Repeat once.

(2) Raise an elbow to the top of your head, forearm dangling behind your head. Grab the elbow with the other hand and pull down toward the back of the neck. Repeat on the other side.

(3) Clasp your hands behind your head. Sitting upright, stretch your elbows backward and hold the stretch.

(4) Sitting upright in your chair, clasp your hands behind your chair back. Straighten your arms as much as possible and raise your hands toward the ceiling.

(5) Reach over your head to the opposite ear. Gently pull your head toward your shoulder; hold for ten seconds, then repeat on the other side.

(6) Roll your shoulders forward, up, back, then down, making the largest circles possible. Repeat in the other direction. These last two stretch the shoulder and neck muscles, which can tighten and cause problems with our arms, as well as cause tension headaches.

(7) Get out of your chair. Our bodies also weren't designed to sit all day. Don't type for more then 30 minutes without taking a break. Get up, stretch, go to your printer, make yourself a cup of tea, or take the dog for a walk. Buy a telephone headset so you can walk around your office while you talk – and you won't have to hold the handset between your neck and shoulder any more

(Summarised from an article by Jeff Johnston in Natural Life newsletter, Nov 94, US$21 from RR1, St George, Ontario, Canada NOE 1 NO, tel & fax 001 519 448 4001.)

'Intensive exercising during actual bouts of backache can help relieve the pain'

- A new treatment for backache which uses intensive exercises during actual bouts of pain has been developed in Denmark. The new approach flies in the face of orthodox medical advice that rest is the best thing for backache. But practitioners say that it can relieve virtually 100 per cent of acute cases and 80 per cent of chronic cases, even in patients who have suffered for years.

'Doctors have always told their back pain patients to keep quiet and warm and not to move – to avoid the things that cause them pain,' says Professor Preben Plum, one of the method's keenest advocates. 'What we do is the exact opposite.' Their exercises are repeated 60 to 100 times during an hour's session. People with acute back pain can only perform these exercises, however, with the help of an assistant – any intelligent, fairly strong adult will do – whose job it is to carry the weight of the sufferer while the movements are made – until he or she feels able to perform them unaided. Most sufferers will feel sufficiently pain-free to start doing the exercises themselves after about an hour, Professor Plum maintains, because by then their back muscles will have started to function normally.

'Back pain is prevalent in our society because machines have taken over most of the work formerly carried out by people'

The treatment, developed by Professor Plum and former bodybuilder Teedy Ofeldt, is based on the theory that back pain is prevalent in our society because machines have taken over most of the work which was formerly carried out by people. This means that many of our muscles, especially those in our backs and shoulders, have become weak and unable to function normally (from the Independent).

• The IT revolution in schools is likely to lead to **back problems** in future – children and adults using computers need **forward tilting chairs** and an angle between head and screen of 20 degrees, according to a report form the Osteopathic Information Service, tel 0118 951 2051 (Sunday Times, Nov 97).

'Between 20 and 80 per cent of children have or will develop back problems'

• Between 20 and 80 per cent of children have or will develop back problems which could affect their skeletal growth and lead to more serious problems in later life. The solutions however are relatively simple: get children to carry their school books in a rucksack; limit the time they spend slouched in front of the TV or computer and try and improve furniture for computers at home and school; get them to take regular exercise; advise them on posture (Anne McHardy in The Guardian, 22/9/98).

'Recumbent workstations reduce back strain'

Alternatives are being sought to the office chairs in which most people spend most of their working lives, and which are thought to be responsible for a rising toll of painful (for the employee) and costly (for the employer) back problems. 'Sitting up straight' may give an employee the correct appearance of studious industry, but it also forces the spine out of its natural 'S' shape into a damaging 'C'.

One means of taking this unnatural stress off the lower spine, currently being explored by a number of furniture designers, is to design 'recumbent' workstations, in which both the worker and the computer they are using can tilt back to an almost horizontal position. Some companies may feel that this is an indecently relaxed posture for their workers to adopt. However, there is evidence that a prone position enhances lateral thinking, so employers might actually benefit from a more creative workforce. Indeed, Thomas Jefferson, probably one of the most energetic and creative souls in human history, designed buildings and ran America from a near-horizontal position, with his legs slightly raised.

Certain senior employees at the BBC, who have to work facing large banks of TV screens, are already using this kind of chair. For the majority of office workers, however, a rather less laid back solution to spine strain is more likely to be introduced. These furniture innovations – such as one company's chest-height conference tables – remove strain on the lower back by requiring one to remain standing (summarised from a story by Steve Connor, entitled 'Chair designers urge office staff to take more laid-back approach' in The Sunday Times).

'Electromagnetic radiation from TVs, mobile phones and computers may trigger asthma attacks and other allergic reactions'

- Scientists from the UK's National Radiological Protection Board have shown that **electromagnetic fields** can damage short-term **memory** in mice and lengthen the time taken to learn tasks. Humans are subjected to electromagnetic fields (at lower levels but for longer periods) from televisions, computers, electrical appliances and power lines (Sunday Times, 29/6/97).
- **Electromagnetic radiation** from TVs, mobile phones and computers may trigger asthma attacks and other allergic reactions, as well as affecting the user's short-term mental abilities (The Times and the Sunday Times, 20/9/98).
- Mobile phone manufacturers, by designing new components which reduce the health risks, seem to be acknowledging the dangers of using a **mobile phone** (The Independent, 25/10/98).
- Mobile phone users – especially heavy users like City traders and Telecom employees – complain of headaches, loss of concentration, skin tingling, burning or twitching, eye tics, poor short-term memory, dementia and

1,001 Health Tips, £6.85 incl. p&p from ISI, 20 Heber Road, London NW2 6AA (tel 0181 208 2853)

fatigue, among other effects, according to Alisdair Philips, a **radiation** expert. "It is too early to say, but we are starting to see **lymphomas** in the neck in heavy phone users. It has been repeatedly shown that a few minutes exposure to cell phone type radiation can transform a five percent active cancer into a 95 per cent active cancer for the duration of the exposure and for a short time afterwards" (The Guardian, 10/11/98).

• Don't wear **bifocals** typing on your computer. You will tilt your head to an unnatural angle and put a strain on your neck, leading to painful **neck problems** (Teleconnect).

• People get tired eyes when staring at **computer screens** because they **blink less** and their eyes dry faster when working on computers. The problem can be remedied by lowering the screen – when people look down rather than straight ahead, their eye openings are smaller, so their eyes dry more slowly (The Times).

• Scientists at Leeds University investigating the problem of radiation-contaminated sheep, have found that feeding them a **fizzy citric acid cocktail** helps lower **radioactivity** (The Independent).

• Bulgarian researchers have found that a grape pigment, **enoviton**, which is present in relatively high concentrations in cabernet sauvignon – the main grape of claret wine – helps the body to excrete **radioactive** substances and makes the immune system better able to fend off the aftereffects of radiation exposure.

• More than 90 per cent of patients with **acrophobia** (a fear of heights) were able to reach target heights after a course of facing these fears in the safe environments of a headset which placed them in a scary **virtual reality** (Alison Goddard in New Scientist, 11/6/94).

• The **Buteyko method**, a new Russian treatment for **asthma** which simply involves learning a new breathing pattern, is now available in Britain.

'The problem asthmatics have is that they breathe too much'

Proponents of the technique, which was developed by the Russian physiologist Professor Konstantin Buteyko, claims that the problem asthmatics have is that they breathe too much. It is well-known that we breathe in oxygen, which passes through the lungs into the bloodstream, and breathe out the waste gas carbon dioxide. Less well-known is the fact that we actually need carbon dioxide in the lungs for the oxygen to pass efficiently into the bloodstream; and that this can be diluted by heavy breathing.

Professor Buteyko tested thousands of asthmatics and found that all of them were over-breathing. The optimum amount is around five litres per minute, but asthmatics were breathing two, three or even four times that amount. The result is that carbon dioxide levels go down and the body responds by constricting the airways – its way of saying, "Stop breathing so much!" The essence of the Buteyko method is that by reducing the level of breathing, the carbon dioxide levels rise and the airways open.

Despite endorsements from prominent asthmatics, including Dr John Stanley of the National Public Health Laboratory, and research which showed 90 per cent of people who tried it reporting improvements and reduced medication, the UK's main asthma organisation, the British National Asthma Campaign, continues to discourage people from trying the Buteyko method. "They say it has not been adequately researched" says Chris Drake, a Buteyko practitioner, "when there has been a double-blind clinical trial in Australia and the interim results have been written up in an Australian medical journal ... They were the best in terms of help for asthmatics ever published."

Chris Drake runs courses in the Buteyko method (£290 for a five-hour course, with a money-back guarantee) at the Hale Clinic, 7 Park Crescent, London W1N 3HE, tel 0171 631 0156, as do The Kingston Natural Healing Centre, 40 Eastbury Road, Kingston KT2 5AN, tel 0181 546 5793. (Summarised from an article by Jerome Burne, entitled 'A shorter intake of breath', in The Independent, 10/6/96.)

- Toners used in **photocopiers** produce dust containing iron, silicon and copper which can cause **lung disease** if inhaled (The Lancet, Sept 96).

- The toxic chemical soup in office air that causes **Sick Building Syndrome** and streaming eyes, sore throats and skin irritations – can be prevented by installing **office plants**: spider plants, tulips, banana plants, philodendrons and lilies are all good at removing specific irritants (New Scientist, 21/6/97).

- Using mulch or **compost** when gardening can cause **organic dust toxic syndrome** (ODTS), with chills, fever and other flu-like symptoms. Precautionary measures include ensuring that the mulch is damp, not dry, so that the dust is contained, using fresh material which has less bacteria, and applying it gently so that minimal dust can be breathed in (Modern Maturity, June 98, monitored by Roger Knights).

- The majority of **greenhouse** workers are sensitive to a microscopic mite that lurks in most greenhouse plants, Tetranychus urticase. This could explain the wheezing, coughing, running eyes and nose of nursery workers or those who spend long hours in a conservatory or greenhouse – the mite can precipitate **asthma**, **hay fever** or **eczema** (Clinical & Experimental Allergy, reported by Dr Thomas Stuttaford in the Times, 8/7/97).

'Fresh cold air with a low water content is better at increasing lung function than the most effective medicines available'

- Fresh cold air with a low water content is the best cure for **asthma**, three to six times more effective in increasing lung function than the most effective

1,001 Health Tips, £6.85 incl. p&p from ISI, 20 Heber Road, London NW2 6AA (tel 0181 208 2853)

74   1,001 HEALTH TIPS

medicines available. House dust mites are one of the chief causes of the asthma epidemic but are not affected by fitted carpets or frequent vacuum cleaning. The sole factor is high humidity. Opening a window for a while is not enough either. In Denmark, mechanical **ventilation**, usually involving at least one complete change of air every hour, can be paid for by the state for severe sufferers (University Hospital, Aarhus, Denmark, reported by David Nicholson-Lord in The Independent, 10/7/92).

• A thirty-second **blast of pure oxygen** will double your recall for several minutes, and the effect will last for 24 hours. These findings were made by Andrew Scholey and Mark Moss, of the University of Northumbria, who conducted blind tests with a sample of volunteers inhaling through a mask for 30 seconds, some of them breathing in oxygen and others ordinary air, (which contains only about twenty per cent oxygen). The participants then listened to series of 15 words, and were asked to recall them six minutes later – at which stage the oxygen-inhalers did twice as well.

'A thirty-second blast of pure oxygen will double your recall for several minutes'

The tests, inspired by the empirical experience of divers and pilots who inhale oxygen at work, provided what is considered conclusive proof that such short blasts improve **short-term memory**, attentiveness and reaction time. They stress that the effect is optimal with inhalation for 30 to 60 seconds. Less or more oxygen than this will do no good and, in the latter case also carries health risks.

The news, however, is not likely to provide much help to cramming students. Scholey maintains that it is neither realistic nor safe to make oxygen more generally available. "The only advice I have is not to revise at the top of a mountain" (summarised from a story by Alison Motluk, entitled 'Oxygen is the stuff of memories', in New Scientist, 21/4/97).

• Drivers instinctively open the car window if they feel drowsy, and **keeping a cool head** should indeed keep people **alert**, according to research by Professor Robert Greene and colleagues at the Harvard Medical School. When your brain heats up (after prolonged exercise and perhaps after prolonged mental activity) 'up go your adenosine levels, firing slows down and the more drowsy and fatigued you feel' (The Independent).

• If motorists would avoid driving when taking certain **tranquillizers** – such as Valium and Mogadon – there could be 1,600 less **traffic accidents**, and 110 fatalities, a year (The Times and The Guardian, 23/10/98).

• Scientists at Lancaster University found a strong statistical link between 'low level' symptoms such as runny nose, headache, red and itchy eyes, breathing problems and lack of energy, and the **volume of traffic** passing close to homes (The Independent).

1,001 Health Tips, *Institute for Social Inventions, London, 1998, 100pp, ISBN 0 948826 50 9*

- To avoid **varicose veins** from too much standing still, people should regularly and rhythmically tighten and relax the leg muscles when standing; and when walking should avoid flipflops and exercise sandals which alter the action at the ankle and the pumping movements of the **calf muscles**; they are also best advised to bath only at night before going to bed to ensure that the heat-dilated blood vessels will not be overstretched by the person standing for long periods (from an item entitled 'Standing Orders', The Times).

- **Wooden kitchen surfaces** are far more **hygienic** than the more modern easy-to-wipe plastic ones, suggests research by Dean Cliver and Nese Ak of Wisconsin University. Whereas bacteria left overnight on a plastic surface multiplies, the natural antimicrobial chemicals which remain in even dead trees enable wooden surfaces to clean themselves ('Looks could kill' in The Economist, monitored for the Institute by Roger Knights).

- A **traumatic memory** can be desensitised by mimicking the **REM** (rapid eye movement) of the most relaxing stage of sleep. At the Mental Research Institute in Palo Alto, California, patients are treated by being asked to follow the repeated quick movements of the therapist's finger while focusing on the traumatic memory (from an unidentified item monitored for the Institute by Roger Knights).

- *Zachariah Evans writes:* Iris Murdoch elegantly describes one of the benefits of sleep as constant refreshment by taking 'little holidays from ourselves'. Unfortunately, we have an infinite capacity for taking things for granted and it is not until we lose the precious 'holidays' for extended periods that we realise the magnitude of the disaster. This happened to me. I became insomniac and unwillingly found myself joined in misery with the other 5 million insomniacs in the UK today. As with many insomniacs, the pills prescribed only made my condition worse; side effects and addiction followed. This wretchedness finally spurred me to invent a cure for the insomnia. A book followed: '**Sleeplessness Cured: The Drug-Free, Quick and Proven Way**'.

I started from the base that insomnia is a disturbing obsession, an aberration of the mind. Necessity was the mother of invention but it had several fathers – philosophers and psychologists among them: from them we know that we can all choose which thought we wish to think; we also all have the power to block out any thought that we do not wish to think. Indeed, it is this blocking process that enables us to think coherently – we can only handle one thought-process at a time.

'Filling the mind with a previously prepared sleep-thought of your choice will block out insomniac thoughts'

As insomniacs know, however, you do not cure yourself simply by deciding not to think the disturbing insomniac thoughts. The mind is immensely

1,001 Health Tips, £6.85 incl. p&p from ISI, 20 Heber Road, London NW2 6AA (tel 0181 208 2853)

powerful, and left with nothing in particular to occupy it the insomnia invasion will certainly return. The innovation was in seeing that, at bedtime, by filling my mind with a previously prepared sleep-thought (my choice) this would block out the insomniac thoughts. As the insomnia could not get in, peace would be restored and sleep would quietly follow. My five nights of commitment to the theory proved it to be a fact. I have never had a bad night since and a survey of my book's readers (two-thirds of them women) found that 6 out of 10 have had success in solving or relieving their insomnia.

'The sleep-thought should concern itself with an intelligent hobby – never day-to-day affairs'

Ideally, the sleep-thought should concern itself with an intelligent hobby – never, never with business or day-to-day affairs. My own hobby is tennis and my sleep-thought is about dates and names of Wimbledon champions. A sleep-thought must be interesting and must be thoroughly learned before attempting to use it in bed. The toughest part is the first two or three nights when the powerful insomnia will try every trick to break in; concentration on the sleep-thought and determination (commitment to the cure) are essential.

Science still doesn't know what sleep and dreaming are for, but from observation of hundreds of insomniacs, I surmise that sleep is not essential for the body to restore itself; it is overwhelmingly the ever-working brain that needs the holidays and it takes these – by dreaming!

(In the book I mention some sleep oddities: perhaps strangest of all concerned a murder that took place on a beach in France. The detective assigned to the case noticed footprints around the body. They proved to be his own; he had himself shot the victim whilst sleepwalking!)

Generally, whatever 'triggers' insomnia, it is the fear of poor sleep that fuels the habit of poor sleep. In essence, my invention replaces a bad habit with a good and effective one. It could save much suffering (and the NHS millions of pounds wasted on sleeping pills) if we were to train lay people in the simple technique of restoring sleep so that they could practise in surgeries and hospitals throughout the country. And as insomnia is a global problem, why not elsewhere in the world?

Zachariah Evans' book Sleeplessness Cured: the Drug-Free, Quick and Proven Way *is available for £3-99 inc p&p from The Insomnia Cure Group, 46 Station Road, Severn Beach, Bristol BS12 3PL.*

• Multiple short **naps** – between twenty and thirty minutes every four hours or so – can reduce total sleep to two to three hours in the 24 for weeks on end without being detrimental to a person's overall performance (adapted from a review by Sheena Meredith in New Scientist, 26/6/93, of 'The 24 Hour Society' by Martin Moore-Ede, published by Piatkus, 230 pages, £18).

• Cancer, hepatitis B and influenza can all be cured by gargling small

amounts of one's own urine, claimed the first World Conference on **Auto-Urine Therapy** (The Guardian).
• Drinking one's **urine** first thing in the morning, if jet-lagged for instance, gives the illusion of a good night's sleep, as urine is rich in **melatonin**, the hormone involved in producing circadian rhythms – according to a study from the University of Newcastle, NSW, Australia. (This is disputed by Surrey University who say that melatonin helps at least two thirds of people suffering from jet lag but is present in urine only in tiny quantities, in its non-active form.) An osteopath in Hertfordshire has been drinking his own urine daily for 20 years and recommends it to patients with asthma, eczema, bad eyesight and other chronic problems.

'Melatonin is said to combat jet-lag, protect cells from free-radicals, boost the immune system, ward off cancer and promote longevity'

• The hormone **melatonin**, secreted naturally in humans but at decreasing levels with age, seems to be emerging as a new panacea. As well as proving very effective as a sleeping pill, the hormone is also said to combat jet-lag, protect cells from free-radical damage, boost the immune system, ward off cancer and promote longevity (Newsweek).
• Many **chronic fatigue syndrome** and ME sufferers have double the **melatonin** levels of non-sufferers, suggesting an overactive immune system, claims a report from Dr Soutzos at Guy's at St Thomas' Hospital (The Independent, 23/6/98).
• The **sleep**-regulating hormone **melatonin** is destroyed in the body by even 15 minutes of light, according to a study led by David Klein at the National Institute of Health in Bethesda. "If you get up in the middle of the night, better leave the light off," recommends the New Scientist summary (7/3/98).
• A technique for improving eyesight, new '**integrated vision therapy**' – where the patient is given a 'visual fitness prescription' (glasses that leave some blur) and is simultaneously encouraged to examine life issues – claims some success (*The Power Behind Your Eyes*, by Robert-Michael Kaplan).
• An American Vision Therapy Clinic claims that its eye-training sessions have helped athletes and those with learning-related visual problems. The Alderwood integration training includes practising focusing on small objects close at hand and in the distance, improving peripheral vision to the sides while looking ahead, and **eye teaming** which helps the eyes work together to focus (The Seattle Times, monitored for the Institute by Roger Knights).
• The recent escalation in cases of acanthamoeba keratitis – rare eye disease caused by a microorganism – may well be explained by the fact that two thirds of **contact lens cleansing solutions** lack hydrogen peroxide, which is the

most efficient chemical in killing the organism (The Guardian).
- One in four **travellers** to the **tropics** may return home with a parasite or **disease** they are unaware of, say doctors from the London School of Hygiene and Tropical Medicine. Tropical travellers should consult their GP for a checkup on their return even if they have no symptoms, they suggest (The Independent).
- If you are stung by a bee, don't worry about whether you should scrape or squeeze out its **sting** – the main thing is that you get it out as **quickly** as possible. This is the conclusion of entomologist Kirk Visscher, who pressed 70 bees against his forearm until they stung him, then waited various lengths of time to remove the stings (The Lancet).
- Alternatively, for the more allergic and fainter of heart, **insect stings** and snake bites can now be removed with a **vacuum pump** developed by the French army and Medicins sans Frontieres. It is available, under the brand name Aspevenin, for £12-49 from larger branches of Boots (The Times).
- A new pill called Program, prescribed by vets, to be given to pets in the spring, rids a household of **fleas**. Dr John Maunder of the Cambridge University Entomology Centre says that 'the pill is sucked up by fleas and a little bit goes into the egg, to such an extent that it never survives. As far as we know, it does absolutely nothing to us or the pets.' (The Times, 21/4/94.)
- Four-legged visitors to the sick and elderly in hospital are being offered a reward – a year's supply of pet food, baskets, collars and other goodies. Armitages, the pet products company, is looking for volunteers to take their dogs or cats to **visit the sick** and elderly once a week. Interested pet owners should contact Fiona Munro on 0602 691692 (The Independent, 28/11/93).
- **Singing** helps keep the palate soft and **prevents snoring**. Snoring often starts once the throat muscles become floppy due to age, lack of exercise or weight gain (Dr Elizabeth Scott, adviser to the Scottish Chamber Orchestra).
- Recent American research reported in the Journal of the National Cancer Institute has shown that prolonged use of **black hair dye** carries with it an increased risk of developing, and dying from, **non-Hodgkin's lymphoma** and multiple myeloma (The Times, April 94).

'One in ten inpatients contracts an infection whilst in hospital'

- One in ten inpatients contracts an **infection** whilst **in hospital** (The Times).
- The discomfort following a **minor accident**, such as knocking one's head or stubbing a toe can be relieved by focusing one's attention in a concentrated way on the injured body part (a tip from a letter to the Institute from Claus Wilcke, Hasenhof 8, 71540 Murrhardt, Germany).

AGEING

- **Large ears** are a good predictor of **longevity**, and a diagonal crease across the earlobe can indicate susceptibility to coronary heart disease (The Times).
- In a study of 7,000 people, daughters born to **older fathers** – those over the age of 50 – were found to live, on average, two years less than those born to younger fathers. It is possible that as people age, their DNA is damaged, and the damage is then inherited by the child (Sunday Times, 15/6/97).

> 'Longevity may be significantly enhanced by eating one third less food than you want'

- Research on a group of rhesus and squirrel monkeys suggests that longevity in humans may be significantly enhanced by eating one third **less food** than you want (American National Institute on Ageing).
- **Thyme** oil, available as 'Efatime' in British health food shops, is thought by some researchers to slow the ageing process. Its high levels of **antioxidants** are thought to protect against the action of free radicals (The Times).
- Older people who take supplements of both **vitamins C** and **E** appear to live significantly longer (Positive Health).
- People over 65 given a daily **vitamin** and mineral supplement were half as likely to suffer infection-related illness, and immune system activity increased (The Lancet, reported in The Independent).
- Elderly patients could soon be advised by their doctors to head for the sun, according to researchers at the University of Delaware. Sick and elderly rats seemed to prefer **hot climates** which induced fevers, and fever is an aid in fighting infection (US News & World Report, 18/5/98).
- Retinoic acid, a derivative of **vitamin A** already used in treatments for acne, may also be effective in mitigating the ageing effects of exposure to the sun (The Times).
- Elderly people, whose bodies are less efficient in freeing **vitamin B12** from food, could benefit from huge supplementary doses of vitamin B12, as could those with pernicious anaemia (Journal of the American Medical Association).

> 'Thyme oil may help slow the ageing process'

- **Zinc** supplements could reduce symptoms of tinnitus and improve **hearing** in the elderly (Alternatives in Health).
- Early tests of a Chinese herbal remedy for **senility** – the dried herb or stem of **Boschniakia rossica** – suggest it may indeed have therapeutic value

---

1,001 Health Tips, £6.85 incl. p&p from ISI, 20 Heber Road, London NW2 6AA (tel 0181 208 2853)

(Positive Health).

- The cell membrane substance **GMI ganglioside** can help to treat some of the symptoms of **Parkinson's** disease by producing the neurotransmitter dopamine which is lacking in Parkinson's sufferers, according to research by Professor Schneider of Thomas Jefferson University in Philadelphia (Daily Telegraph, 23/6/98). Other recently approved drugs which appear to slow the dopamine decline in Parkinson's sufferers include: Tasmar (tolcapone), and Requip (ropinorole) and Miramex which both mimic dopamine.
- A glass of **cranberry juice** may halve **urinary tract infection** rates in elderly women. Cranberries contain proanthocyanidins, a compound which can stop bacteria attaching itself to the urinary tract (Rutgers University, New York, reported in The Guardian, 3/11/98).
- Very high doses of **vitamin A**, if prescribed early enough, may provide a cure for age-related macular degeneration (ARMD), a very common cause of **blindness in the over-50s**. The minimum effective dosage is currently being researched, since too much vitamin A can damage the liver (New Scientist).
- **Prayer** helped people regain health according to the South Medical Journal which investigated the 'therapeutic effect of intercessory prayer in a coronary health unit' (Harry Schultz newsletter).
- While **daily praying**, Bible study or weekly churchgoing can help to **lower blood pressure**, exposure to religious radio or TV programmes can increase it, according to a study of 4000 elderly North Carolinians (Time, 24/8/98).
- Research into the mysterious **DHEA hormone**, produced by the cortex of the adrenal gland, by Dr Samuel S.C. Yen at the University of California in San Diego, suggests it may have a role to play in mitigating the effects of ageing. In a small study of 16 middle-aged to elderly people who received either DHEA or a placebo for a year, Dr Yen saw a 75 per cent increase in overall wellbeing among those receiving the hormone. At a Washington conference in June 1995, he reported that his subjects coped better with stress, got around more easily and slept better. Men, but not women, also gained muscle and bone and lost body fat, although neither reported a change in libido.

Dr Marc R. Blackman, chief of endocrinology at Johns Hopkins Bayview Medical Centre, added that other research had pointed to important effects of DHEA on cardiovascular function and the risk of heart disease, especially among men, and on immune function, which normally declines significantly with age.

> **'Men, but not women, gained muscle and bone and lost body fat, although neither reported a change in libido'**

There are a few nay-sayers among hormone cognoscenti about stoking the healthy elderly with hormones. For example, Dr Clemmons of the University of North Carolina pointed out that like all drugs, hormone treatments had side effects, although the risks would be more acceptable in people who have a lot to gain.

Pregnenolone is the other precursor hormone that some advise taking alongside DHEA. William Regelson MD in his book 'The Super-Hormone Promise' (published by Simon & Shuster, ISBN 0 684 83011 6) extols pregnenolone as potentially a memory enhancer and a treatment for arthritis and for depression. Steven Fowkes, editor of 'Smart Drug News' says in the March 96 edition of 'Intelli-Scope that 'Dr Eugene Roberts [has observed] that even minute quantities of pregnenolone as small as a few hundred molecules have a very potent effect on the ability of mice to learn and navigate mazes ... I think the risks [with DHEA and pregnenolone] are minimal when you're dealing with replacement dosages, ie, less than the amount your body would produce if it were healthy.' The introduction to this interview with Steven Fowkes says that there has been a recent paper indicating that 'patients receiving DHEA supplements slept better, had more energy and were better equipped to handle stress compared to the placebo group not receiving the DHEA.'

Using a Web search engine to find references to DHEA will bring up several thousand items about its effects and the details of a number of firms where you can order by credit card. Many references, such as those above, make it sound like a too-good-to-be-true wonder drug, reversing ageing, preventing cancer and heart disease and restoring libido. Others point to a theoretical risk of triggering hormone-responsive cancers ('DHEA changes the colour of rodent livers from pink to brown; when 16 rats were fed DHEA for a year and a half, in a recent study at Northwestern University, 14 developed liver cancer.'). Go to http://www.naples.net/~nfn03605/dheafaq.htm for answers to frequently asked questions. See also www.raysahelian.com/dhea.html for the dangers.

For ordering pregnenolone and DHEA by e-mail, one of the cheaper sources seems to be New Way International of 4705 Oxbow Road, Rockville, MD 20852—2311, USA (tel 301 468 8836; e-mail: newway@erols.com) who sell, for instance, a minimum quantity of 120 slow release 25mg capsules of pure DHEA (with a maximum recommended dosage of 2 capsules a day) for $23.90 (postage $4.50 USA or $10 internationally by air, with the package arriving in the UK, for instance, seemingly without problem, labelled 'dietary supplement'). Several of the web references stress that the DHEA should be of the slow release microcrystalline non-wild-yam derived kind.

(Summarised from various sources including an article by Jane E. Brody in The New York Times, 18/7/96, monitored by Nicholas Saunders.)

The Attitude Factor

Thomas Blakeslee's innovatory book, The Attitude Factor – Extend your life by changing the way you think, *is published by Thorsons (1997, ISBN 0 7225 3546 5, 239 pages, £7.99) and won the 1998 Health Social Innovations Award. Here is the Institute for Social Inventions' introduction to (and summary of) this important work – readers are referred to Blakeslee's book and website for the full story.*

• A radical Internet experiment replicates **longevity research** from Germany which demonstrated that a healthy mental attitude is a far better predictor of long life than a healthy lifestyle. The book's associated website (www.attitudefactor.com) provides people with tests for their wellbeing, sense of pleasure and self-regulation. It also provides a tailor-made set of exercises to help people improve their attitudes in these departments.

'The Attitude Factor – extending your life by changing the way you think'

By following up those tested in future years, to see who are still alive and well, Blakeslee hopes to be able to test the wider applicability of the findings from Germany.

By extending, internationalising and popularising this Heidelberg research, Blakeslee's work could revolutionise the way society approaches education, health promotion and treatment of the elderly, whilst greatly increasing people's sense of happiness and wellbeing. There are very few other individuals in history for whom the same claim could be made.

'Blakeslee's work could revolutionise the way society approaches education, health promotion and treatment of the elderly'

The following questions and tests are adapted excerpts from Blakeslee's website and book, although readers are urged to treat what follows as a mere taster and to complete the full tests at www.attitudefactor.com and to follow the full set of exercises in his book.

Thomas Blakeslee

About three hundred of the people in self-regulation experiments organised by Dr Ronald Grossarth-Maticek in Heidelberg had good scores on self-regulation but very unhealthy lifestyles. For at least ten years, these people smoked 20 or more cigarettes a day and drank over 60 grams of alcohol a day. They also had an unhealthy diet and did little exercise. In spite of their unhealthy lifestyles, this group outlived a group with healthy lifestyles but poor self-regulation by 8.5 years. Clearly self-regulation has a health impact which is stronger than and goes much deeper than just health habits. Healthy lifestyle was defined in this experiment as no smoking or drinking, good diet and at least 1.5 hours of exercise a day.

> 'These people smoked 20 or more cigarettes a day and outlived a group with healthy lifestyles, but poor self-regulation, by 8.5 years'

Q: What is the purpose of the Attitude Factor book and website?

To develop and prove the effectiveness of a new way to improve health and lengthen life by identifying and correcting unhealthy mental habits. These techniques were developed and experimentally proven by Dr. Ronald Grossarth-Maticek in the above-mentioned experiments using elderly residents of Heidelberg, Germany.

> 'Feelings of pleasure and wellbeing originate in the ancient, nonverbal parts of the brain that we share with lower animals'

Because the results were so spectacularly successful, they have been ignored or greeted with scepticism by the medical profession. By taking the tests on the website and using the corrective materials offered, you can improve your own health prospects and at the same time help us to repeat the amazing improvements in health and lifespan in the original experiments. By replicating these experiments in a way that can't be ignored, I hope that we can finally convince the medical establishment of the supreme importance of mental factors in promotion of good health.

Q: Why are feelings of pleasure and wellbeing so important to good health?

Feelings of pleasure and wellbeing originate in the ancient, nonverbal parts of the brain that we share with lower animals through our common evolutionary past. This part of the brain also interacts with body systems which control blood pressure and immune responses. When your basic needs are met, your body's systems work at peak efficiency.

When these same needs are frustrated, you may have chronic feelings of hopelessness which drive your body's systems into a kind of 'self-destruct mode' where diseases and cancer can easily get a foothold and heart disease, strokes and accidents become more likely. Your ability to think logically in words is a powerful ability which also has the power to ruin your health if it is directed at goals which are actually at odds with your basic needs.

Q: What is self-regulation?

1,001 Health Tips, £6.85 incl. p&p from ISI, 20 Heber Road, London NW2 6AA (tel 0181 208 2853)

84   1,001 HEALTH TIPS

Self-regulation means that you regulate your behaviour to maximise long-term pleasure and wellbeing. It means that you pay attention to the results of your behaviour and make corrective adjustments as needed. Regulation is what a thermostat does when it regulates the temperature in a building by turning on the heater only when it is too cold. If the thermostat breaks, the regulation breaks down and the building gets hotter and hotter. Similarly, when self-regulation breaks down, habitual behaviours which produce poor results are simply repeated endlessly.

'Self-regulation means regulating your behaviour to maximise wellbeing, making corrective adjustments as needed'

The result of such behavioural ruts is as disastrous as when the thermostat breaks. In both cases, failure to adjust response to outcomes causes things to get worse and worse. Scores on the self-regulation test are very accurate predictors of future health because people who are good at self-regulation are able to maximise their long-term pleasure and wellbeing.

Q: Isn't the idea of maximising pleasure and wellbeing the same as hedonism?

Good self-regulation emphasises long-term happiness. The negative connotation of hedonism is usually associated with dissolute behaviour that produces bad long-term consequences such as overweight, addiction, debts, etc. Relaxing is good for you, but doing nothing all day soon results in bad consequences. The important thing is to develop a healthy balance that maximises your long-term pleasure and wellbeing.

Q: Why is the immune system disabled by feelings of hopelessness?

Evolution works by culling the weak and preserving the strong. Mating battles in some species allow only the strongest to reproduce. Predators cull the weak in others. Perhaps the weakening of the human immune system by feelings of helplessness is nature's way of culling the outcasts and the unsuccessful to improve the breed.

'The probability of dying was doubled in the week after losing a mate'

One massive study in Finland examined the health records of 96,000 widowed people and found that their probability of dying was actually doubled in the week after losing their mate. Feelings of pleasure and wellbeing are messages from the ancient parts of your brain and limbic system that you are thriving and your immune system is running at peak efficiency. Feelings of hopelessness indicate the opposite.

Q: Why haven't I heard about this research before?

1,001 Health Tips, *Institute for Social Inventions, London, 1998, 100pp, ISBN 0 948826 50 9*

The unfortunate separation of physical medicine from psychology has caused this important work to be largely ignored by the medical establishment. Part of the problem is that the work was reported in respected psychological journals which are not read by doctors. Another problem is that the results are so amazingly strong that many people dismissed them as 'too good to be true'.

'Today's entire medical paradigm needs to be rethought; but doctors are reluctant to accept paradigm-upsetting information'

The problem is that the entire medical paradigm of today needs to be rethought and doctors are reluctant to accept anything that so upsets their sense of understanding. Denial has always been a common defence against paradigm-upsetting information.

Q: Who is Dr Grossarth-Maticek?

Dr Grossarth-Maticek has been doing research on the connection between mental factors and health since the early 60s. He created both of the tests used in the Attitude Factor book and website. He also created and proved the effectiveness of a new kind of corrective therapy designed to improve health prospects by teaching healthy mental habits. The amazing effectiveness of this therapy will hopefully be duplicated by the programs on the website.

Q: Have Dr Grossarth-Maticek's experiments been replicated?

The large scale and long duration of these experiments is unprecedented. There have been several less ambitious experiments that have achieved results which support the validity of Grossarth-Maticek's conclusions. The long time required to test results probably prevents most researchers from undertaking such experiments.

'Dr Grossarth-Maticek spent over a million dollars of family money on his research'

Dr Grossarth-Maticek spent over a million dollars of family money on his research. The Attitude Factor website greatly reduces the cost of gathering data by automating it and eliminating the need for paid interviewers making house calls. In five to ten years' time I hope to be able to report that this automated method is equally effective in predicting and improving health prospects.

Q: Where and when will your research results be published?

In five to ten years' time I plan to compare the test scores gathered by this site with health status as determined by public records. I will also compare the health status of people who complete our one-year self-improvement programme with those who don't take it. The health effect of a careful reading of my book The Attitude Factor will also be determined. The report of these results will be submitted to a major medical journal such as the British Medical Journal.

A pleasure and wellbeing test linked to longevity

In 1973, Dr Ronald Grossarth-Maticek's assistants gave a pleasure and wellbeing test to some 3,055 elderly residents of Heidelberg, Germany. The 15-question test, reproduced below, measures how intensely and how often you experience feelings of pleasure and wellbeing.

'30 times more likely to be alive and well'

21 years after the test was given, the health status of the people who had taken the test was checked and it was found that those who had scored highest on the test were 30 times more likely to be alive and well than those who had low scores. This amazing correlation between feelings of pleasure and wellbeing and later good health tells us that being happy is truly more than a luxury. It's a matter of life and death.

Instructions: Answer each of the following questions by circling one of the seven numbers. Answer with complete honesty and with a long-term focus. Try to ignore your present mood and answer the questions honestly based on your usual feelings over the years and, in particular, the past 12 months:

1. How intensely do you feel pleasure? (For example, from love, contentment, sexual pleasure, foods, sports, nature, music, etc.).
Slight: 1 / 2 /3 / 4 / 5 / 6 / 7 Intense

2. How long do your feelings of pleasure last when they do occur?
Seconds 1 / 2 (minutes) / 3 / 4 (hours) / 5 / 6 (all day) / 7 (days)

3. How often do you get feeling of pleasure? (while doing sports, sleeping, having sex, listening to music, working, joyfully fulfilling your needs, etc)
Almost never 1 / 2 (monthly) / 3 / 4 (weekly) / 5 / 6 / 7 Daily

4. Do you sacrifice your short-term pleasure when necessary to avoid negative consequences or improve your prospects for pleasure in the long-term?
Never 1 / 2 / 3 / 4 / 5 / 6 / 7 Always

5. Are you afraid of your own feelings of pleasure, particularly in areas of great emotional importance such as love?
Total fear 1 /2 /3 / 4 / 5 / 6 / 7 No fear

6. How certain are you that you will feel pleasure in the future?
Impossible 1 / 2 / 3 / 4 / 5 / 6 / 7 Certain

7. Do you believe that the highest peak of pleasure you have felt in your life will ever be equalled or surpassed in the future?
Unlikely 1 / 2 / 3 / 4 / 5 / 6 / 7 Certain

8. When you feel a sense of wellbeing, how strong is the feeling?
Blocked 1 / 2 / 3 / 4 / 5 / 6 / 7 Powerful
9. How long do your feelings of wellbeing last when they occur?
Seconds 1 / 2 (minutes) / 3 / 4 (hours) / 5 / 6 (days) / 7 Almost continuously
10. How frequently do you experience a feeling of wellbeing?
Almost never 1 / 2 (monthly) / 3 / 4 (weekly) / 5 / 6 (daily) /7 Many times a day
11. Do you sacrifice your short-term wellbeing when necessary to avoid negative consequences or improve your prospects for wellbeing in the long term?
Never 1 / 2 / 3 / 4 / 5 / 6 / 7 Always
12. When a feeling of wellbeing occurs, do you sometimes act in ways that destroy it?
Almost always 1 / 2 / 3 / 4 / 5 / 6 / 7 Almost never
13. How strong is your feeling of security that you will experience wellbeing in the future?
Unlikely 1 / 2 / 3 / 4 / 5 / 6 / 7 Certain
14. Do you believe that the strongest feelings of wellbeing that you have experienced in the past will be felt again in the future?
Unlikely 1 / 2 / 3 / 4 / 5 / 6 / 7 Certain
15. After you have experienced pleasure do you often have negative feelings such as guilt, bad conscience, depression or physical symptoms?
Almost always 1 / 2 / 3 / 4 / 5 / 6 / 7 Almost never

Scoring: Divide total of all numbers circled by 15.

In the Heidelberg experiment, the percentage of people alive and well 21 years later included:
Only 2.5 per cent of the people with scores of 2 or less
30 per cent of those with a score of 4.1 per cent
41 per cent of those with a score of 5.1 per cent
51 per cent of those with a score of 5.6 per cent
75 per cent of those with scores of 6.5 per cent or better.

Note too that a study by Bacon, Remeker and Ertler (Psychosomatic Medicine 14, 1952: 453-60) of 40 women with breast cancer found that only 5 were freely capable of orgasm. 25 had never experienced orgasm and considered sex a distasteful wifely duty, 5 were still virgins and 5 had orgasms only rarely.

Test for anti-emotional behaviour

Way back in 1965, as part of one of his early studies which led to his theories on self-regulation, Dr Grossarth-Maticek's interviewers questioned 1,341 elderly residents of Crvenka, Yugoslavia about their personality, health habits and attitudes. In 1976, when they checked the people's health status, they found that 11 of the questions relating to rational and anti-emotional behaviour had been amazingly predictive of future ill-health. In fact, 158 of the 166 cancer deaths were among those people who had answered yes to 10 or all 11 of the questions below:

'158 of the 166 cancer deaths were among those people who had answered yes to 10 or all 11 of the questions'

1. Do you always try to do what is reasonable and logical?
2. Do you always try to understand people and their behaviour, so that you seldom respond emotionally?
3. Do you try to act rationally in all interpersonal situations?
4. Do you try to overcome all interpersonal conflicts by intelligence and reason, trying hard not to show any emotional response?
5. If someone deeply hurts your feelings, do you nevertheless try to treat him rationally and to understand his way of behaving (so that you hardly ever attack and deprecate him or treat him purely emotionally)?
6. Do you succeed in avoiding most interpersonal conflicts by relying on your reason and logic (often contrary to your feelings)?
7. If someone acts against your needs and desires, do you nevertheless try to understand him?
8. Do you behave in almost all life situations so rationally that only very rarely your behaviour is influenced by emotions only?
9. Is your behaviour frequently influenced by emotions to such a degree that from a purely rational point of view it would have to be regarded as nonsensical or detrimental?
10. Do you try to understand others even if you do not like them?
11. Does your rationality prevent you from attacking others, even if there are sufficient reasons for doing so?

The people who answered yes to 10 or 11 of these questions were also 10 times more likely to die of heart attacks or strokes. Completely ignoring your own needs and feelings appears to be a very unhealthy habit. Logical thinking is extremely powerful, but like many powerful things it is capable of doing serious damage when used improperly. Notice that bad health came only to those who carried rationality to the extreme. Considering other people's feelings to some degree is healthy because your happiness is increased when people like you. A balance between taking care of your own feelings and considering others results in a 'middle' score. The really destructive pattern seems to be when you never consider your own feelings.

1,001 Health Tips, *Institute for Social Inventions*, London, 1998, 100pp, ISBN 0 948826 50 9

'Childhood experiences, such as trying to keep the peace in a chaotic family, often teach people to suppress their own feelings'

Childhood experiences, such as trying to keep peace in a chaotic family, often start people down a path where they learn to suppress their own feelings. Good health requires that your verbal self learns to trust and act on the important feedback from your feelings. It must nurture them and respond to them, not suppress them.

The risk catalogue

Every time you boldly face a minor risk it builds your confidence and feelings of being in control. Fearful attitudes can shorten your life. Let's look at the numbers. The insurance industry and safety engineers have developed extensive tables of the actual risks in your life. Your calculated life expectancy can be determined by subtracting the Loss of Life Expectancy numbers below (expressed in days) from your basic life expectancy as determined by your age and sex. For example, if you spend one year pursuing a hang-gliding hobby, take 25 days off your life expectancy.

Reduced life expectancy catalogue
The numbers indicate the total number of days of life expectancy lost. A negative figure indicates the number of days gained

Smoking, 2 packs/day men 3139
Smoking, 1 pack/day men 2409
    women 1533
Passive smoking 50
Cardiovascular disease 2043
Cancer, all 1247
Breast cancer 109
Pulmonary disease 164
Pneumonia 103
All accidents 366
Motor vehicle 207
    collisions 87
    pedestrians 36
Home 74
    falls at home 13
Overweight 25 per cent 1303
    per per cent point 52
Unemployment 500

Air travel 3.7
Ocean travel 33
Occupation (average) 60
    Agriculture 320
    Mine, quarry 167
    Construction 227
    Manufacturing 40
    High-wire act 100
    Professional diving 500
    Championship auto racing 100
Sports/year of participation:
    Professional boxing 8
    Hang gliding 25
    Mountain climbing, all 10
    dedicated 110
    Mountain hiking 0.9
    Parachuting 25
    Sail planing 9
    Scuba diving, amateur 7
    Skiing-racing 0.5
    Snowmobiling 2
    Bicycling 6
Air pollution 77
Pesticide residue, food 12
Hazardous wastes 4
Contaminated drinking water 1.3
AIDS 50
Medical radiation 6
Natural radiation 9
Radon gas in homes 29
Hurricanes 0.3
Tornadoes 0.8
Excess heat 0.7
Lightning 11
Floods 0.4
Earthquakes 0.2
Tsunami 0.15
Weather related accidents 1.8
Venomous plants, animals 0.5
    snakes, lizards, spiders 0.08
    hornets, wasps, bees 0.4
Dog bites 0.12
Injury by animals 0.6

Ageing

Poor social ties 1642
Good social ties -1642
Pleasure score of 3 5000
Pleasure score of 4 3760
Pleasure score of 5 -1606
Pleasure score of 5.5 -2732
Self-regulation score 2 2737
Self-regulation score 3 766
Self-regulation score 4 -803
Self-regulation score 5 -4781

If you really want to improve your prospects for a long, healthy life, 'attitude jogging' is the fruitful place to direct your efforts. The risk numbers clearly show that your attitude factor, as reflected by your scores on the attitude tests, has a much greater potential for adding years of good health and happiness to your life than all of the tiny risks people worry themselves about put together.

'If avoiding second-hand smoke is limiting your social life, you are certainly shortening your life by trying to lengthen it'

Notice, for example, that good 'social connections' can make a 3,285-day (9-year) difference in your life expectancy. If avoiding second-hand smoke (50 days) is limiting your social life, you are certainly shortening your life by trying to lengthen it.

Just being married makes a 1,825-day (5-year) difference in your life expectancy. If you were offered a pill that would add five years to your life with no bad side-effects, wouldn't you take it without hesitation?

Attitude jogging

Here is a sample selection from the hundreds of exercises that Blakeslee suggests for improving your attitude factor:

'Next time a friend invites you to do something challenging, say yes, and then push through any temptations to find excuses to cancel'

Make a list of things you used to enjoy in your youth.
Make a commitment pact with a close friend or lover to help each other work on attitudes.
Try foods at an ethnic restaurant which you have previously avoided

---

1,001 Health Tips, £6.85 incl. p&p from ISI, 20 Heber Road, London NW2 6AA (tel 0181 208 2853)

because you consider the food 'creepy'.

Count your laughs for a whole day. A researcher found that small children laugh an average of 450 times a day, while adults average only 50.

Watch the video of Two for the Road with Audrey Hepburn and Albert Finney. The contrast between joyfully living as back-packers in their youth and their present fussing about luxury hotel conditions vividly demonstrates what Attitude Jogging is all about.

Next time a friend invites you to do something challenging, say yes and then push through any temptations to find excuses to cancel or drop out.

Does drinking alcohol give you pleasure and improve your ability to communicate your feelings? If the answer is yes, pour yourself a drink and enjoy!

'If you live alone, think how you could share your accommodation with a good friend'

People are social animals. If you are currently living alone, think how you could share your accommodation with a good friend or relative.

Volunteer to work on some kind of useful cause where you can directly help others.

Dance to music with no thought of how you look. Let your body naturally express its response to the music.

Thomas Blakeslee, 101 California Avenue #701, Santa Monica, CA 90403, USA (tel 001 301 393 9686; fax 395 4706; e-mail: TBlakeslee@attitudefactor.com; web: www.attitudefactor.com).

Alzheimer's

- Lee Glickstein in his book *Be heard now* says:

I gave a talk to a Veterans' Administration programme for elderly women caring for their disabled husbands – and my subject was laughter.

'He forgets who I am and proposes marriage. I love it. We laugh and laugh'

I asked in hopeful desperation, "Do any of you have examples of how you have used humour to cope with your situation?"

A 70-year old woman named Catherine shot up her hand. She stood up and said, "My husband and I have always laughed a lot and still do. He has Alzheimer's Disease. Every morning he sort of forgets who I am and proposes marriage. I love it. We laugh and laugh."

One by one, the women shared their poignant, funny experiences.

The theme was clear: only with laughter could they survive. I haven't

spoken to a more cheerful, inspirational group since.
(Summarised from Be heard now! – How to compel rapt attention every time you speak, *by Lee Glickstein, Leeway Press, 450 Taraval Street #218, San Francisco, CA 94116, USA; 1996; $16.50; ISBN 0 9653322 33).*

• **Anti-inflammatory drugs** (NSAIDS) such as ibuprofen and naproxen, often prescribed for arthritis, and carrying significant side-effects such as ulcers, do nevertheless appear to halve the risk of Alzheimer's disease, according to an American study (The Times).

• Those taking nonsteroidal **anti-inflammatory drugs** such as ibuprofen, indomethacin and even aspirin, appear less likely to contract Alzheimer's (Nigel Hawkes, The Times, 6/2/95).

'Sweden with its high fish and low fat diet has the lowest incidence of Alzheimer's'

• Researchers believe that a **low-fat diet** may reduce the risk of Alzheimer's. Sweden with its high fish and low fat diet has the lowest incidence of Alzheimer's (Time, 30/6/97, monitored for the Institute by Roger Knights).

• Alzheimer's sufferers could delay the onset of the disease with **B12** supplements and **folates**, claim researchers at the University of Oxford (New Scientist, 24/10/98).

• Those with the equivalent of A levels or **university degrees** were up to three times less likely to suffer dementia in old age (British Medical Journal).

• Prof. Brian Austen of St George's Hospital, London, has shown that raised **blood cholesterol** may be a factor in some cases of Alzheimer's. Exercise, low-fat diet and outdoor pursuits could help protect people from the disease (The Times, Dec 97).

• 27 per cent of Alzheimer's patients, who took **ginkgo biloba** (extracted from the bark, nuts and leaves of the maidenhair tree) in a study by the New York Institute for Medical Research paid for by the drug's manufacturers, showed improvements in mental functioning, as against 14 per cent in the placebo group (Thomas Maugh II, Los Angeles Times, 22/10/97, monitored by Roger Knights).

'Ginkgo biloba extract improved cognitive performance and social functioning in outpatients with mild to severe dementia'

• 120mg of a standardised **ginkgo biloba** extract given to outpatients with mild to severe **dementia** for one year proved successful in improving their cognitive performnce and social functioning, preventing or relieving symptoms such as memory loss, difficulty in concentrating, tiredness, anxiety, and headaches. Ginkgo has already been used by doctors in the treatment of circulatory problems (Health Guardian, June 98).

- High doses of **vitamin E** modestly slow the progress of Alzheimer's, working about as well as the more costly selegiline, according to a study by Mary Sano and colleagues at Columbia University (Seattle Times, 24/4/97, monitored for the Institute by Roger Knights).
- **Vitamin E** supplements appeared to slow the rate of physical decline in patients with Alzheimer's disease. Since the patients studied were already suffering from the disease, it is unclear whether the vitamin might have a preventative effect (New England Journal of Medicine, April 97).
- However, vitamin E **supplements** may actually reduce the body's reserves of the vitamin, since they contain only one of its two forms. Both forms are needed to receive its health benefits, but high doses of the form found in most supplements will actually deplete reserves of the second (New Scientist).
- A long-term Oxford University study of 250 dementia patients has shown that the blood samples of those with Alzheimer's tend to reveal a diet low in the **vitamins B6, B12** and **folic acid** (Steve Connor, Sunday Times, 26/4/98).
- The cold sore virus, **herpes simplex**, which often migrates to the brain, has been linked to the development of Alzheimer's disease in the 30 per cent of people whose brains also contain the protein Apoe e-4 (The Lancet).
- Nicotine and **nicotine-like drugs** can protect brain cells from Alzheimer's-induced deterioration, claim a team from Duke University in North Carolina. Their aim is to develop drugs which act like nicotine, and attach themselves to the acetylcholine receptors on the brain cell surface, but which are non-addictive and without harmful side effects (The Times, 12/11/98).
- Against the grain of recent medical wisdom, a Dutch study of Alzheimer's disease suggested that **smokers** had double the risk of contracting the disease, and retained an increased risk even after giving up (New Scientist).
- A postmortem study has found that more than half the drivers over 65 killed in **car accidents** have some, very possibly undiagnosed, form of Alzheimer's disease (The Times).

'Galathamine, found in daffodils, shows great promise in the treatment of the symptoms of Alzheimer's'

- **Daffodils** contain a chemical called galathamine, which shows great promise in the treatment of the symptoms of Alzheimer's disease (The Times).
- A Newcastle research team is investigating the potential of **sage oil** to alleviate **memory loss** associated with Alzheimer's disease (New Scientist).

1,001 Health Tips, *Institute for Social Inventions, London, 1998, 100pp, ISBN 0 948826 50 9*

- Research suggests that **fathering** a child in one's mid-30s or upwards doubles its risk of developing **Alzheimer's** disease in later life (British Journal of Psychiatry).
- Low **linguistic sophistication** is, from an early age, an effective predictor of Alzheimer's. A study of a closed community of nuns showed that women whose writing style in their twenties had displayed 'idea density' and 'grammatical complexity' were much less likely to contract the disease in later years. Conversely, those who had had a simpler way with words at the same age were much more susceptible – implying, say the researchers, a strong genetic component in the disease (The Times).
- Rats that exercised had much higher levels of brain-derived **neurotrophic** factor – a factor reported to decline with the onset of Alzheimer's (Dr Carl Cotman, University of California).
- **Zinc** may help trigger Alzheimer's – although a deficiency can cause slow wound healing and loss of sense of taste amongst other problems. In 1992, the University of Melbourne gave zinc supplements to five Alzheimer's patients but within four days their cognitive decay markedly accelerated (David Steel, The Wall Street Journal, 2/9/94).
- A BBC Panorama programme was accused of scaremongering by linking **mercury** in dental fillings with Alzheimer's Disease. Dr Boyd Haley's work, featured in the programme, linked mercury even at low levels in the brain with Alzheimer's (The Times, 19/7/94).

'Old people with very small heads were 14 times more likely to show signs of Alzheimer's'

- Old people with very **small heads** were 14 times more likely to show signs of Alzheimer's and other forms of age-related dementia than those with large heads (Dr Amy Graes of the Battelle Centre for Public Health Research in Seattle).
- People with big heads or, more exactly, **large brains**, appear to be less vulnerable to the deterioration associated with Alzheimer's disease (Ms. London).

'Moderate wine consumption of around three to four glasses a day reduced the risk of Alzheimer's by 75 per cent in a study of over-65s'

- Moderate consumption of **wine**, equivalent to around three to four glasses a day, has been confirmed as reducing the risk of developing Alzheimer's disease by 75 per cent in a French study of over-65s. Neither light (one to two glasses a day) nor heavy drinking (upwards of four) appear to carry the same benefits (Neurological Review).

• The nicotonic receptor plays a role in neuroprotection. Administering nicotine to a damaged animal brain helps it recover much faster. This backs up the notion that **nicotine** prevents degeneration in Alzheimer's disease, according to research reported in New Scientist (9/10/93, page 14). 'Nicotine significantly improved attentional and information processing abilities of patients with Alzheimer's disease' (a letter to The Times from Dr Gemma Jones of the Institute of Psychiatry, London). Smokers have a reported 50 per cent reduced risk of developing Alzheimer's.

• Adding **silicon** to drinking water could reduce the risk of Alzheimer's disease according to Derek Birchall, Professor of Inorganic Chemistry at the University of Keele. 'If further work establishes the link between silicon and Alzheimer's disease, there would be a very strong case for areas deficient in silicon to be raised to the same levels as those in the south of England and Kent' (The Independent, Ann Barrett).

• Alzheimer's could be **spread by coughing**, according to researchers from Wayne State University in Detroit. Postmortem studies of the brains of Alzheimer sufferers found 17 out of 19 of them infected with the microbe Chlamydia pneumoniae which is spread by sneezes and coughs (The Guardian, 13/8/98).

• **Drugs** which could help Alzheimer sufferers in the future include: rivastigmine (exelon) and galantamine (reminyl) – possible memory boosters; metrifonate (bilarcil) – which may slow down the development of symptoms; and memantine – which may help with the ability to perform daily tasks (National Enquirer, 3/11/98, monitored for the Institute by Roger Knights).

Arthritis

• **Fasting** is known to be an effective treatment for rheumatoid arthritis, but most patients relapse on reintroduction of food. The effect of fasting followed by one year of a vegetarian diet was assessed in this randomized, single-blind controlled trial.

'Fasting followed by a vegetarian diet eases arthritis'

27 patients were allocated to a four-week stay at a health farm. They began with a seven to ten day subtotal fast – taking only herbal teas, garlic, vegetable broth, decoction of potatoes and parsley, and juice extracts from carrots, beets and celery. After the fast the patients reintroduced a 'new' food item every second day. If they noticed an increase in pain, stiffness or joint swelling within

two to 48 hours this item was omitted from the diet for at least seven days. If symptoms were exacerbated on reintroduction of this food item, it was excluded from the diet for the rest of the study period. During the first 3.5 months, the patients were asked not to eat food that contained gluten, meat, fish, eggs, dairy products, refined sugar or citrus fruits. Salt, strong spices, and preservatives were avoided – likewise alcoholic beverages, tea and coffee. After this period, the patients were allowed to reintroduce milk, other dairy products and gluten-containing foods in the way described above. The patients who did not use cod liver oil supplemented their diet with vitamin D during the first four months.

'Gluten, meat, fish, eggs, dairy products, sugar, citrus fruits, salt, spices, preservatives, alcohol, tea and coffee are avoided initially'

A control group of 26 patients stayed for four weeks at a convalescent home, but ate an ordinary diet throughout the whole study period.

After four weeks at the health farm the diet group showed a significant improvement in the number of tender joints, Ritchie's articular index, the number of swollen joints, pain scores, the duration of morning stiffness, grip strength, erythrocyte sedimentation rate, C-reactive protein, white blood cell count and a health assessment questionnaire score.

In the control group, only pain score improved significantly. The benefits in the diet group were still present after one year, and evaluation of the whole course showed significant advantages for the diet group in all measured indices.

Food allergy or intolerance is unlikely to explain the improvement in all the patients who changed their diet. Interest has been drawn to dietary fatty acids and their ability to modulate the inflammatory process (Kremer JM, Lawrence DA, Jubix W, et al. 'Dietary fish oil and olive oil supplementation in patients with rheumatoid arthritis. Clinical and immunological effects.' Arthritis Rheum 1 1990; 33: 810-20). A switch to vegetarian diet causes an extensive change in the profile of the fatty acids of the serum phospholipids. These changes may favour production of prostaglandins and leukotrienes with less inflammatory activity.

This dietary regimen seems to be a useful supplement to conventional medical treatment of rheumatoid arthritis.

'Controlled trial of fasting and one-year vegetarian diet in rheumatoid arthritis' by Jens Kjeldsen-Kragh, Margaretha Haugen, Christian F. Borchgrevink, Even Laerum, Morten Eek, Petter Mowinkel, Knut Hovi, Oystein Forre. Dr J. Kjeldsen-Kragh is at present at the Institute of Immunology and Rheumatology, National Hospital, Olso, Norway, tel 47 2 867010; fax 47 2 207287. (Adapted from an article in the Lancet, 12/10/91, by Dr Jens Kjeldsen-

Kragh and colleagues of the Department of General Practice, University of Oslo, and from a report in the Independent by Celia Hall.)

'Rheumatoid arthritis sufferers were twice as likely as non-sufferers to have had close contact with cats between the ages of 10 and 15'

• A US study showed that sufferers from rheumatoid arthritis were more than twice as likely as non-sufferers to have had close contact with **cats** between the ages of 10 and 15 (US News & World Report, monitored for the Institute by Roger Knights).

• Jobs that involve repeated knee-bending, squatting or climbing stairs increase the risk of **osteoarthritis**, according to a study at the Medical Research Council's environmental epidemiology unit in Southampton (The Independent).

• Those with osteoarthritis of the knee should wear **trainers** with good shock absorption, to reduce the load on the knee when the heel strikes the pavement (Prof. Dieppe at Bristol University, reported in The Times by Hether Kirby).

• **Shoes** should be adequately cushioned in the heel and weight should be kept down, so as to avoid **plantar fasciitis**, increasingly severe pain under the heel bone which is normally worst in the morning (Dr Stuttaford, Times, 24/7/97).

• 50 grams of **fresh ginger** every day can inhibit two of the enzymes responsible for inflammation in arthritis (Odenske University in Denmark).

• **Mobic**, the first in a new generation of anti-inflammatory drugs for arthritis, has far fewer unpleasant side-effects than its predecessors (The Times).

• The following **herbs** have exhibited anti-inflammatory effects: Articulin-F, Reumalex, Devil's Claw, Feverfew and the Tripterygium wilfordi root (Proof, 1998).

'Cherries or blueberries may be helpful for both rheumatoid and osteo-arthritis'

• Half a pound of fresh cherries or **blueberries** per day may be helpful for both rheumatoid and osteoarthritis, since they contain proanthocyanidins that aid in collagen metabolism and decrease joint inflammation (Positive Health).

• Dr Jasson Theodosakis claims in his book *The Arthritis Cure* (St Martin's Press, $22.95) that replacing **glucosamine and chondroitin**, two substances produced naturally by the body, can "slow, halt or prevent the degeneration of cartilage". Time magazine (17/2/97, 'The Arthritis Cure?' by Geoffrey Cowley) reports that test tube studies do indeed suggest that glucosamine can stimulate cartilage production, while chondroitin slows its removal. Both nutrients are safe even at high doses. A combination capsule called **cosamin** is sold by Nutramax, a Baltimore company, who say that many vets are using a similar product to treat animals.

• The **antibiotic minocycline** (used to treat acne) can have dramatic effects against rheumatoid arthritis, if used early in the course of the disease, according to researchers at the University of Nebraska (Reuters, 10/11/97).

'green-lipped New Zealand mussel preventing neutropolis from causing inflammation and helping relieve symptoms of arthritis'

• Biologists from the University of Auckland have identified a glycoprotein in the green-lipped New Zealand mussel (on sale as **seatone** in health food shops in the UK) which blocks the action of neutropolis (white blood cells which allow attacks on healthy tissue), thus preventing neutropolis from causing inflammation and helping relieve symptoms of arthritis (New Scientist, 30/4/94).

• A non-toxic treatment which involves giving patients orange juice mixed with **purified collagen** extracted from chicken cartilage and bone alleviates the symptoms of rheumatoid arthritis, according to David Trentham and fellow rheumatologists at Beth Israel Hospital and the Harvard School of Medicine. The collagen molecules seem to migrate to the joints, secreting a hormone-like substance which tones down the white blood cell attack on the patient's own collagen (Robert Cooke in The Guardian, 25/9/93).

1,001 Health Tips, £6.85 incl. p&p from ISI, 20 Heber Road, London NW2 6AA (tel 0181 208 2853)

AND FINALLY...

Health advice online

• If you want to find out more about any of the subjects in this book, the Internet (available at most main libraries) is the best source for free health information. The information, however, is often highly unrealiable, particularly on websites selling pills and medicines. From amongst the myriad of health sites, here are some recommendations:

Medline is very comprehensive, providing free access to abstracts of recent medical research papers on every topic under the sun, using a simple search procedure – go to <www.healthy.net/library/search/medline.htm>.

For general medical information with an American slant try Medscape at <www.medscape.com>.

For access to information on cancer try: <www.oncolink.upenn.edu>.

About 70 online cancer information and support groups are to be found via: <www.medinfo.org>

For over 250 searchable health and medical newsgroups go to: <www.medexplorer.com>.

A recently launched website <www.DrKoop.com> rates the 12,000 plus health sites on the web. Former US Surgeon General Koop is a patients' rights advocate, whose site offers disease and drug information.

Twelve warning signs of health

• Twelve warning signs of health
(1) Persistent presence of support network.
(2) Chronic positive expectations; tendency to frame events in a constructive light.
(3) Episodic peak experiences.
(4) Sense of spiritual involvement.
(5) Increased sensitivity.
(6) Tendency to adapt to changing conditions.
(7) Rapid response and recovery of adrenaline system due to repeated challenges.
(8) Increased appetite for physical activity.
(9) Tendency to identify and communicate feelings.
(10) Repeated episodes of gratitude, generosity or related emotions.
(11) Compulsion to contribute to society.
(12) Persistent sense of humour.

From a bulletin board in Waldport, Oregon, unidentified author, reprinted in Whole Earth Review *(Winter 94).*

INDEX

A
abortions 15
accidents 78
acne 11
acrophobia 72
acupuncture 21, 49
addiction 60, 61
aerobics 67, 68
ageing 5, 19, 49, 66, 67, **79**, 80
Aids 27, 28
alcohol 5, 17, 20, 21, 27, 39, 40, 47, **52**, 53, 72, 83, 95
alcoholism 54, 55
alertness 74
aluminium 66
Alzheimer's 18, 59, 93, 94, 95, 96
anafranil 6
anal seepage 52
anger 9
ankylosing spondylitis 68
antibiotics 22, 33, 59, 99
antioxidants 21, 28, 34, 46, 48, 49, 50, 79
antiperspirants 66
anxiety 10, 57, 60, 64
appetite 49, 52
apples 47, 50
arguments 66
arteries 36
arthritis 45, 61, 81, 93, 96, 98; *see also* rheumatism

aspirin 22, 24, 28, 57, 93
asthma 33, 34, 36, 47, 50, 51, 57, 59, 72, 73
atridox 26
Attitude Factor 82
aubergines 41
autism 37, 39, 60
avocado 8
ayahuasca 60

B
back 69, 70
baldness 5, 7
bananas 22, 25
barbecues 44
beds 33
bees 78
beer 39, 40, 52
bergamot oil 25
betacarotene 21, 46, 48, 49
bicycle 8
birth 11
    Caesarian 12;
    companion 12;
    birth control pill 11;
    defects 14; at home 12; premature 11, 12, 14
Blakeslee, Thomas 82
bleeding 57
blindness 49, 80
blinking 72
blood 22; clots 10; pressure 64, 80
blueberries 98
bones, brittle 66
brain 52, 54, 57, 65, 66, 67, 95
bran 14, 40, 41
bras 15
bread 28, 42, 59
breakfast 41, 49
breast cancer; *see cancer, breast*
breast milk 35
breastfeeding 17, 35
breathing 26, 74
brittle bones 66
broccoli 16
brussels sprouts 46
Buteyko method 72
butter 42

C
cabbage 45
caffeine 47
calcium 16
cancer 5, 11, 13, 16, 1, 24, 28, 44, 45, 46, 47, 48, 49, 50, 53, 58, 66, 76, 77, 81, 88, 100; bladder 45; bowel 40, 57; breast 11, 14, 15, 16, 18, 19, 43, 46, 67; colon 10, 18, 40, 43, 48, 53, 57, 67; gastric 46, 50; lung 21, 43, 46, 50; oral 39, 53; prostate 6, 7, 8; rectal 18; skin 25, 45, 48; stomach 44, 48; testicular 7, 67; uterine 10, 19
cannabis 11, 59

carbohydrates 68
carrots 42, 48
casein 39
cataracts 28
cathechins 48
cats 14, 98; *see also pets*
celery 25
chairs 70
chaparral 57
chemotherapy 16, 59, 68
cherries 98
chewing gum 26, 36
children 31, 70
chocolate 39
cholesterol 41, 42, 45, 52, 94
chondroitin 98
chronic fatigue syndrome 66, 77
circumcision 34
cocaine 61
coffee 11, 13, 24, 36, 47
colds 39, 47, 59, 65
collagen 99
combretastatin 58
comfrey 57
compost 73
computers 71, 72
conception 11
constipation 14, 40, 66
coronary artery disease 44
cosmetics 6
cot death 34
coughing 96
cranberry juice 80
creativity 64, 67
Crohn's disease 44

D

daffodils 95
dandruff 33
daylight 10
delinquency 36
deodorants 66
depression 10, 21, 49, 50, 60, 64, 81
dermatitis 32
detergents 6
DHEA 80
diabetes 36, 41, 45, 48
diarrhoea 36
diet 39, 48, 49, 50, 57, 68, 79, 83, 97
dogs 24; *see also pets*
domination 6
drugs 57, 61; *see also alcohol & smoking*
dyspraxia 36

E

ears 36, 67, 79; earache 36; *see also tinnitus*
eating 39, 41, 48, 52, 60
ecstasy 60
eczema 33, 35, 73
egg donors 11
ejaculation, premature 6
electromagnetic fields 71
emotions 88
ephedra 57
epidural 58
estrogen 19
evening primrose oil 17, 45
evista 19
exercise 7, 9, 10, 14, 22, 23, 42, 67, 68, 69, 82
eyes 77, 80

F

fasting 41, 96
fats 22, 23
fathers 79
fenfluramine 60
fertility 6
fever 79
fibre 40, 41, 46, 48
finasteride 5
fish 10, 14, 22, 27, 28, 36, 42, 44, 45, 46, 93
flavonoids 47, 50
fleas 78
flu 65, 76
fluoride 26
folic acid 12, 26, 66, 94
food 39, 79
friends 65
fruit 10, 26, 42, 43, 50
fruit juices 27, 36, 49, 52, 80, 99
fungal infections 58

G

gallstones 53
garlic 45, 96
gelatine 42
genistein 48
germander 57
ginger 45, 98
ginkgo biloba 94
glaucoma 59
glucosamine 98
gluten 39
glycine 47
gout 53
grains 51

grape juice 52
greenhouses 73
Grossarth-Maticek, Dr 85
gum disease 12, 26
gymnastics 36

H

haemorrhoids 14, 52
hair 5, 6, 7, 78
hair dye 78
hands 5
hangover 52
hay fever 33, 57, 73
headache 20
headband 20
heads 95
health; advice online 100; warning signs of 100
hearing 79; see also ears & tinnitus
heart 5, 9, 12, 18, 22, 23, 24, 28, 34, 39, 42, 43, 44, 46, 47, 50, 52, 53, 65, 79, 80, 89
hepatitis B 76
herbs 57, 79, 98
heroin 61
herpes 48, 95
hiccups 51
hip 66
HIV 27, 28
hormones 6, 7, 14, 15, 19, 81; see also HRT
hospital 78
hot dogs 32
HRC Detox Formula 55
HRT 5, 17, 18, 19
hunger 49
hyperactivity 52
hypnosis 21

I

ibogaine 61
ibuprofen 93
immune system 32, 39, 48, 51, 53, 58, 65, 66, 67, 77, 79, 80, 85
impotence 9, 46
infertility 11
injections 37
insomnia 75; see also sleep
intelligence 6, 18, 37
internet 100
iodine 51
iron 23, 45

J

jaundice 34
joss-sticks 32

K

kidney 16
kissing 29
kitchen 75
kiwi fruit 46
knee-bending 98

L

labour 13
laughter 53, 92
lemons 19
leukaemia 32
licorice 45
life expectancy 90
lifestyle 64
linseed oil 46
liver 57
lobelia 57
longevity 5, 37, 77, 79, 82; see also ageing
Lotsof, Howard 61
low-fat diet 93
lung 35, 73; see also cancer, lung
lustral 10
lycopene 7, 46

M

ma huang 57
magnesium 46, 50
margarine 41, 42
marijuana 11, 59
massage 20, 66
MDMA 60
ME 66, 77
meat 14, 42, 43
meditation 31
Mediterranean diet 42
Medline 100
melanoma 24
melatonin 15, 77
memory 18, 41, 52, 71, 74, 75, 81, 95
men 5, 79
menopause 5, 15, 17, 18, 19; see also HRT
menstruation 10, 15
mercury 95
midrid 20
migraines 20, 60
milk 14, 17, 19, 26, 35, 39; breast 51
minerals 54
miniskirts 10
Mirror Image Therapy 29
miscarriage 13, 35
mistletoe 28
mobile phones 71
mouthwash 53
Multiple Sclerosis 59
music 13, 41
mussels, green-lipped 99

N

naps 76
nasal decongestants 9
neck 72
neoprene sports shorts 10
nicotine 95, 96
night 44
nipples 15
nitroglycerin 52
non-Hodgkin's lymphoma 78
nu-trim 41
nuts 5, 42, 43

O

obesity; *see weight*
olive oil 42
onions 47
optimists 65
orange juice 16, 99
oranges 22
organic 6
osteoarthritis 98
osteoporosis 19, 24, 36, 44, 45
overweight; *see weight*
oxygen 74
oxytocin 17

P

Parkinson's Disease 28, 59, 80
pelvic floor exercises 9
peptic ulceration 53
pessimists 65
pesticides 32
pets 36, 64, 78; *see also cats & dogs*
photocopiers 73
plantar fasciitis 98
plastics 6
pleasure 84
PMT 10, 60
pork 43
potassium 22, 46
potatoes 51
prayer 80
pregnancy 11, 12, 13, 14
pregnenolone 81
premature birth 11, 12, 14
premenstrual; see *PMT*
prostate 8; enlargement 8; prostatitis 7; *see also cancer, prostrate*
prozac 60
psoriasis 25

Q

quinine 16

R

radioactivity 72
rape seed oil 44
REM 75
repetitive strain injuries 69
rheumatism 17, 28, 68, 96, 98, 99; *see also arthritis*
risks 90
royal jelly 51
running 36, 67, 68

S

SAD 10
sage oil 95
sandwiches 32
saunas 12
saw-palmetto 8
schizophrenia 35, 46, 47, 64
seatone 99
secretin 39
selenium 5, 8, 27, 34, 45, 46
self-regulation 84
serotonin 46, 47, 60, 66
sex 6, 8, 11, 14, 17, 65, 81; *see also impotence*
shampoo 33
shark cartilage 45, 58
shoes 75, 98
shyness 65
Sick Building Syndrome 73
silicon 96
singing 78
skin 19, 24, 48; *see also eczema*
sleep 75, 76, 77, 81
slipped disks 53
smell 7, 24
smoking 9, 13, 21, 34, 68, 83, 91, 95
snoring 9, 78
soy sauce 44
soya 6, 7, 44, 45, 48, 66
spanking 37
spectacles 72, 77
sperm 5, 6, 9
spices 45
spinach 22, 43, 48, 49
spine 36
sporta 36, 67, 91
St John's Wort 17, 49, 50
sting 78
stress 11, 37, 53, 65, 66, 81
stretching 68
stroke 22, 23, 49, 57, 59, 89; *see also heart*
students 65
sudafed 57

Index

sugar 14, 51
sun 23, 25, 79
surfactants 6
swimming 26, 37

T

tea 11, 24, 47, 48
teabags 48
teeth 12, 18, 20, 22, 26, 27, 36
television 37, 71
temperature 12
testosterone 5
therapy 64; group 16; magnet 50; Mirror Image Therapy 29
theratope 16
throat 40; *see also cancer, oral*
thrush 59
thyme 79
thyroid disease 51
tin cans 13
tinnitus 20, 79
tomatoes 7, 22, 46
tongue 26
toothpaste 26
toxic waste 13
toxoplasmosis 14
traffic 74
trainers 98; *see also shoes*
tranquillizers 74
triclosan 26
tropical diseases 78

U

ulcers 59
ultrasound 12
umbilical cord 14
unemployment 32
urinary tract infection 80
urine 47, 77, 80

V

varicose veins 14, 75
vasectomy 29
vegetable oils 8
vegetables 10, 22, 40, 42, 43, 45, 48, 49, 50, 51, 97
vegetarians 43, 97
ventilation 65, 74
virtual reality 72
virus 28, 66
vitamins 54; vitamin A 14, 32, 45, 79, 80; B group 12, 21, 26, 46, 47, 79, 94; C 16, 23, 34, 39, 40, 45, 46, 48, 50, 67, 79; D 16, 23; E 6, 23, 45, 46, 48, 50, 79, 94;
vodka 52, 53

W

walking 23, 36
warts 58
washing 33
washing powders 6
water 6, 35, 40, 42, 49, 96
weight 6, 13, 15, 49, 60, 93
wellbeing 83
whisky 52, 53
willow bark 57
wine 19, 27, 39, 40, 47, 52, 53, 72, 95
winter 10, 65
women 10
wood 75
wrinkles 19, 42; *see also ageing*

Y

yeast 59

yoghurt 49
yohimbe 57

Z

zinc 32, 45, 79, 95

1,001 Health Tips, £6.85 incl. p&p from ISI, 20 Heber Road, London NW2 6AA (tel 0181 208 2853)

Institute publications available

This form can be photocopied or orders can be placed by phone (with credit card and with a small supplementary charge) or by letter (with cheque from a UK-based bank in £s sterling).
• **I wish to be sent the following ticked PUBLICATIONS** - (P & p included. 10% off for Institute subscribers, except for those books marked [*])

[*] '**The New Natural Death Handbook**', cheap, green and d-i-y funerals, Good Funeral Guide to undertakers, caring for the dying at home, living wills, woodland burial grounds. £11-65. Or from Natural Death Centre direct.
[*] '**Natural Death & Woodland Burials**', people's tips and advice. Complements the Handbook. £5.95, 1998. Or from the Natural Death Centre direct.
[*] '**Sooner Or Later**', preparing for dying and family-organised funerals, a supplement to the Natural Death Handbook. £5-95, 1997. Or from Natural Death Centre direct.
[*] '**Creative Endings**', creative ways of approaching dying and funerals, £5-95, 1996. Or from Natural Death Centre direct.
[*] '**Poem for the Day - 366 Poems, Old and New, Worth Learning By Heart**', with foreword by Wendy Cope. 400 page book with a poem for each day of the year. £11-49. Or from Natural Death Centre direct.
• '**Time Out Book of Country Walks**' by Nicholas Albery. A walk for each Saturday from a station near London, plus a Saturday Walkers Club, £10-99.
• '**Creative Speculations**', provocative ideas, foreword Brian Eno, £14.85.
• '**DIY Futures**', 250 new social tools and incentives, £14-85.
• '**The Book of Visions, An Encyclopedia of Social Innovations**', foreword by Anita Roddick; a 352 A4 page compendium of best ideas and projects. £18-49 (£20-65 from abroad by credit card).
• '**The Forest Garden**' by Robert Hart. How to establish a Forest Garden, in town or country, consisting entirely of fruit and nut trees and bushes, wild and self-seeding vegetables and herbs. £3-25. 3rd edition.
• '**Alternative Gomera - Guide to a fortnight's walking round Gomera Island near Tenerife**' by Nicholas Albery, 3rd Edition. £8-85. Map £5-50 extra.
• '**Re-Inventing Democracy**'. Designs for more responsive, yet more stable, governance by David Chapman, advance price £8-95 (£13-95 libraries & institutions). To be published '98 or '99.
• '**The Neal's Yard Story**', full of useful ideas for small businesses and urban renewal. £1-95.
• '**The Solution for South Africa**', an influential cantonisation scheme, as a way of avoiding ethnic turmoil in South Africa. £7.

Institute publications

- **'Social Invention Workshops - A Manual for Use in Schools'**, used by the Institute in its school workshops. £2-50.
- **'Future Workshops - How to Create Desirable Futures'**, by Robert Jungk, used by groups throughout Europe as a manual. £8-85.
- **'The Problem Solving Pocketbook'**, an overview of all the main ways to solve problems, plus some wild ones. £2-95.
- **'Opening the Mind's Eye'**, by Margaret Chisman. Group exercises on themes such as truth, beauty and goodness, designing new commandments, etc. £2-50.
- **'Being True to Yourself'**, by Margaret Chisman, completes her trilogy of exercises for groups. These ones encourage insight and self-understanding. £4-95.
- **LOGO for Windows**. Fun software plus game for learning maths and programming. £25 (software item). £45 (multi-machine licence).
- **'Auction of Promises - how to raise £16,000 in one evening'**, by Kara Conti, for church, school and community groups. How to auction off services such as 4 hours' massage, computer consultancy etc. £1-95.

- Enclosed is £15 for an Institute **subscription**. Pay by UK Standing Order if possible, in which case £1 off: £14. (Outside UK £17 by credit card.)
- (Alternatively and at no extra charge) I wish to apply for **membership**, and enclose £15 (outside UK £17 by credit card) and details of profession, skills and interests, and of socially innovative projects or ideas.
(£1 off above £15 fee for those who pay by UK banker's order - fill in form below. Members and subscribers receive the book-length Annual in the summer - *state if you want this year's or next year's* - plus often a booklet from the Natural Death Centre, and 10% off most Institute publications, except those with [*]. They can also apply to join walks near London every Saturday and Salon discussions.)
- I also wish to make a **donation** and enclose £..... / I am prepared to offer my services as a volunteer / or to send socially inventive cuttings from enclosed list of publications.
- I enclose a card (and address) of **friend** to whom these goods are to be sent. Outside UK:
- 10% extra for sea-mail postage, 50% extra if wanting airmail on books.

Outside UK, unless paying by credit card or by UK cheque or UK cash notes, you must add:
- £3-50 (if paying by foreign or Irish cash notes, for bank charges).
- £10 (if paying by foreign cheque - even from Eire - for bank charges).
- No extra if paying UK sterling by bankers draft **with bank charges paid your end**: (to Institute for Social Inventions account, bank number 60 13 34, account number 38843803, bank address: National Westminster Bank, 298 Elgin Avenue, London W9, UK).

1,001 Health Tips, *£6.85 incl. p&p from ISI, 20 Heber Road, London NW2 6AA (tel 0181 208 2853)*

108   1,001 HEALTH TIPS

Payment by credit card: please add 4.2% for the bank's fee, unless otherwise stated. We accept any non-Switch card with American Express, Eurocard, Mastercard or Visa logos. By e-mail, phone, fax, letter, give your card-holder number, expiry date, registered address, name and initials & signature. This is the cheapest way to pay from outside UK.

NAME (caps) ....

ADDRESS..

....

....

TEL. No..
Please return this form with cheques payable to: '**Institute for Social Inventions**', 20 Heber Road, London NW2 6AA, (tel 0181 208 2853; fax 0181 452 6434; e-mail: rhino@dial.pipex.com).

━━━━━━━━━━━━━━━━━━━━━━━━━━━━━━

UK STANDING ORDER FORM - please fill in and return to Institute for Social Inventions, 20 Heber Road, London NW2 6AA. USE CAPITALS.

MY BANK..
BANK ADDRESS..

....

MY ACCOUNT NO. ....
Please pay to the Institute for Social Inventions £........ **annually**, starting on the ...... day of .... 19....... (or as soon after this date as possible). Their account is bank number 60 13 34, account number 38843803, bank address: National Westminster Bank, 298 Elgin Avenue, London W9, UK.

NAME (caps) ....

ADDRESS..

....

TEL. No..
SIGNATURE...
DATE..

1,001 Health Tips, *Institute for Social Inventions, London, 1998, 100pp, ISBN 0 948826 50 9*